Partial Seizure Disorders

Help for Patients and Families

Mitzi Walt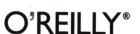

O'REILLY®

Beijing • Cambridge • Farnham • Köln • Paris • Sebastopol • Taipei • Tokyo

Partial Seizure Disorders: Help for Patients and Families
by Mitzi Waltz

Copyright © 2001 O'Reilly & Associates, Inc. All rights reserved.
Printed in the United States of America.

Published by O'Reilly & Associates, Inc., 101 Morris Street, Sebastopol, CA 95472.

Editor: Nancy Keene

Production Editor: Catherine Morris

Cover Designer: Terri Driscoll

Printing History:

February 2001: First Edition

Library of Congress Cataloging-in-Publication Data:

Waltz, Mitzi
    Partial seizure disorders: help for patients and families / Mitzi Waltz.
        p. cm.—(Patient-centered guides)
    Includes bibliographical references and index.
    ISBN 0-596-50003-3
    1. Epilepsy--Popular works. I. Title. II. Series.

This book is printed on acid-free paper with 85% recycled content, 15% post-consumer waste. O'Reilly & Associates, Inc., is committed to using paper with the highest recycled content available consistent with high quality.

[M]

To Jerod

Table of Contents

Preface

THIS BOOK IS INTENDED to bring together all of the basic information needed by people diagnosed with a partial seizure disorder and by parents of children who have these forms of epilepsy. Professionals who work with this population should also find this book useful.

The first two chapters provide a broad overview of epilepsy in general, and of partial seizure disorders in particular. Subsequent chapters cover lifestyle issues, topics specific to children, treatment options, dealing with insurance problems and the healthcare system, and more. Appendix A, *Resources*, lists books, web sites, organizations, and special diagnostic and treatment centers to help you find additional information that meets your needs. Contact information for all organizations mentioned in the book can be found in this appendix. Appendix B, *Seizure Diary*, is a reproducible form for keeping track of seizures and associated events, which may help you gain greater insight into and control over your symptoms. The *Glossary* is a mini-dictionary of terms associated with seizure disorders and their treatment. When documents or studies are referenced in the text with footnotes, full citations can be found in the *Notes* section.

Partial seizure disorders occur in both males and females, so we've tried to alternate between pronouns when talking about patients, as well as healthcare professionals.

We've done our best to provide accurate information about resources in the English-speaking world, including North America, the UK, the Republic of Ireland, Australia, and New Zealand. Seizure disorders are a universal phenomenon, however, and occur in all races and nationalities. Readers in other parts of the world may be able to find local resources and current information in languages other than English on the World Wide Web: some of the web sites and email discussion groups listed in Appendix A of this book can point you toward resources in your part of the world. Simply because we are writing in the US, some information will be skewed toward American readers. Most, however, will be useful to all.

Throughout the text we present findings from the latest medical research. This information is not intended as medical advice. Please consult your physician before starting, stopping, or changing any medical treatment, including changing your diet and trying other alternative health practices. Some of the health information provided comes from small studies or is controversial in nature. We don't endorse any particular medical or therapeutic approach to seizure disorders, and we encourage readers to carefully examine any claims made by healthcare facilities, pharmaceutical firms, supplement manufacturers, therapists, and others before implementing new treatments.

This book is not just about the science of partial seizure disorders; it also covers the personal experience of living with these conditions. It blends technical information with stories from adults and children who have partial complex seizures and stories from the people who love them. These quotes are offset from the rest of the text and presented in italics. In their quotes, people with first-hand knowledge share their emotions, experiences, thoughts, and coping methods. In some cases, names and other identifying details have been changed at the person's request.

Acknowledgments

Many people with epilepsy and parents of children with epilepsy took the time to answer questions about their medical histories and lives, speaking from the heart on topics ranging from diagnosis to brain surgery. They deserve much of the credit for this book, as their replies guided its structure and contents. I would particularly like to express my appreciation to Cherilyn Cox, Robert Jon Daisher, Beth Fausnaugh, Robert Gill, Becky Iremonger, Ron Jensen, Mary Lowe, Iain MacNaughton, Jacky (Jacqueline) Madine, RN, Patricia A. Murphy, Vicki Hill Riedel, Barb Reisinger, Jacque Rogers, Maria Sansalone, Rebecca Stevenson, disability advocate Ken Wilkinson, and C. Wilson.

EPILEPSY-L, an online mailing list for people with all types of seizure disorders, kindly allowed me free access to a large group of persons around the world who live with these challenges every day. Participating in their conversations gave me a window into their lives, from the joys of finding a medication that works, to the pain of job discrimination. I thank them for answering my questions with candor and patience and commend them for creating such a caring community.

The manuscript of this book was reviewed before publication by Paul Garcia, MD, associate professor of neurology at the University of California, San Francisco and a clinician at the Northern California Comprehensive Epilepsy Center; Anthony Murro, MD, associate professor of neurology and director of the EEG Laboratory at the Medical College of Georgia; psychologist Frank Feiner, PhD; Dion Graybeal, MD, assistant professor in neurology at the University of Texas Southwestern Medical Center in Dallas; Doug Hyder, MD, of the University of Southern California and Children's Hospital Los Angeles; Pat Murphy, editor of the "Epilepsy Wellness Newsletter;" family member Chuck Toporek; and parent Wendy Dowhower. Their comments, criticisms, suggestions, and corrections have made this a much better book.

The Epilepsy Foundation has also been a primary and extraordinarily valuable resource. Created by people with epilepsy, this organization gives voice to the concerns of individuals and families affected by seizure disorders. It works in the nation's legislatures, in the media, online, in its excellent annual conferences, and in state and local chapters to provide information, help, and hope.

Nancy Keene, Linda Lamb, Shawnde Paull, and all of the extraordinarily professional editorial and production staff at O'Reilly & Associates have my utmost respect and admiration, as does my literary agent, Karen Nazor.

Thanks to Nancy Keene (again), Wendy Hobbie, and Kathy Ruccione. Some of the material in Chapter 3, 4, and 7 was adapted from their book *Childhood Cancer Survivors: A Practical Guide to Your Future* (O'Reilly & Associates, 2000).

I would also like to thank my friends Jerod Poore and Vicki Hill Riedel for piquing my interest in this project. Your travels down this road have not been easy, but they've definitely helped to educate me. I hope that this book will pass that gift on to many others.

Despite the inspiration and contributions of so many, any errors, omissions, misstatements, or flaws are entirely my own.

—Mitzi Waltz

If you would like to comment on this book or offer suggestions for future editions, please send email to *guides@oreilly.com*, or write to O'Reilly & Associates, Inc. at 101 Morris St., Sebastopol, California, 95472.

CHAPTER 1

Introduction to Partial Seizure Disorders

PARTIAL SEIZURE DISORDERS are forms of epilepsy that involve a specific part of the brain rather than the entire brain. Symptoms can vary widely: some patients have no physical signs at all, experiencing only mental or sensory changes during a seizure, while others may experience numbness, shaking, or involuntary movements of one or more body parts. This book focuses on simple partial and complex partial seizures, including temporal lobe epilepsy.

This chapter covers both common and uncommon symptoms of partial seizure disorders. It will explain what's known about the causes and signs of these conditions, and review brain anatomy as it relates to seizures. Many seizure-related terms and concepts are also introduced to help you better understand your doctor and your medical records.

Recognizing partial seizures

Partial seizures can sometimes be hard to recognize. People who experience partial seizures may have trouble explaining their symptoms or be reluctant to talk about them. Because some people with partial seizures never have convulsions, doctors may not first consider epilepsy as a possible explanation for their symptoms.

Here are some descriptions of real people who had puzzling symptoms, and who were later diagnosed with a partial seizure disorder:

* For years, 11-year-old Jake's teachers have complained that he's often "spaced out" in class. Lately he's been reporting terrible headaches and stomachaches, too. Could these symptoms be connected?

* Joseph just got fired...again. He's 23 years old and burns through jobs quickly. Every now and then he erupts in rage for seemingly no reason

at all, in inappropriate settings, and with little memory of what happened when the episode is over. His rages are embarrassing and puzzling for Joseph and his family, especially since they don't seem to be connected to events or frustrations. They don't even seem purposeful—indeed, he can't communicate during an episode, even though his words and actions make it look like he's boiling mad about something.

- Cory is 40 years old. She regularly experiences sudden, disabling episodes of dread—without warning, and without relationship to any inner experiences or anything happening around her. Often the feeling is followed by a buzzing sound in her ears and strange physical symptoms that she has trouble putting into words. She feels as though her mind separates from her body during these odd episodes.

- Eight-year-old Billy is a conundrum. He has episodes that look like mild seizures, but three EEGs have found nothing. His symptoms wax and wane, and include smelling, hearing, and seeing things that aren't there, staring off into space, and making odd movements with his mouth and left arm. A neurologist has suggested that he has "psychosomatic seizures," but his parents don't agree. They don't think a grade school child would know how to fake these symptoms.

Although Jake, Joseph, Cory, and Billy had very different symptoms, each was actually experiencing partial seizures. Not everyone with symptoms like theirs has a seizure disorder, of course, but it is one explanation that deserves attention—and in the case of these people, it turned out to be the correct one.

What is a seizure?

Seizures can be compared to an electrical storm in the brain. A seizure begins in a damaged or malfunctioning area of the brain called a seizure focus. The seizure focus might be a tiny lesion or scar caused by high fevers in childhood, lack of oxygen at or before birth, damage from a virus, or a previous head injury. Some people are probably born with the potential to have seizures, which may or may not ever be activated.

Anyone can have a seizure under certain conditions. The most common reasons for having a single seizure are a high fever (especially in infants and children), sleep deprivation, or a reaction to certain drugs or medicines.

Having a single seizure does not indicate that a person has a seizure disorder or epilepsy.

Epilepsy is defined as repeated episodes of seizure activity. About one percent of all people have epilepsy, but many more will have a single seizure at some time in their life. Seizures occur when a person's seizure threshold—the brain's tendency to allow seizures to start and spread—is abnormally low. Around 40 different types of seizures or seizure disorders have been identified. Many of these are listed and defined in the *Glossary* at the end of this book.

When a seizure begins in a single area of the brain, it's called a partial seizure. When seizure activity starts simultaneously in many different areas of the brain, it's called a generalized seizure. Partial seizure disorders are more common, and paradoxically less well known, than is epilepsy with generalized seizures.

Partial seizures are further divided into simple partial and complex partial seizures. Although simple and complex partial seizures usually do not look dramatic to other people, they can have serious consequences for patients who have them. The physical and emotional effects of partial seizures—dissociation, loss of coordination, memory loss, fatigue, mood swings, and physical pain, among others—can make them very difficult to live with.

If left untreated, seizure activity may become more severe. Seizures may happen increasingly often or be more difficult to control. When seizures last for more than 30 minutes, there is a possibility of permanent brain damage in some cases.

The four most common types of seizures are described in the following list:

- **Simple partial seizures.** These events (also known as focal cortical seizures) do not cause a person to lose consciousness. They usually include some kind of repetitive body movement, such as an eye flutter or a shaking arm or leg.

- **Complex partial seizures.** These events include impairment, but not necessarily loss, of consciousness. Complex partial seizures are also called psychomotor seizures, and they include the temporal lobe seizures that characterize a specific seizure disorder known as temporal lobe epilepsy (TLE).

- **Tonic-clonic seizures.** These events occur when aberrant electrical activity spreads throughout multiple areas of the brain, affecting a person's physical control as well as her mental state. Tonic-clonic seizures are also known as generalized seizures, convulsions, or fits. They were once called grand mal (French for "very bad") seizures. In some cases, a tonic-clonic seizure may begin with a partial seizure. (See "Auras: A type of simple partial seizure," later in this chapter.)

- **Absence seizures.** These events also affect large areas of the brain, but without causing convulsions—instead, it's as if the conscious mind switches off temporarily. A person having an absence seizure may simply sit and stare. He will be unresponsive if spoken to, may drop things, and may make some small, repetitive movements. Absence seizures were formerly called petit mal (French for "not so bad") seizures. Some people mistakenly use this older term to describe complex partial seizures as well.

Usually seizure disorders are chronic problems, but they can normally be controlled to some degree with medication and lifestyle adjustments. Occasionally a preventable cause can be identified for a seizure disorder, such as a medication that has artificially lowered a person's seizure threshold. Eliminating that cause may also eliminate the seizures.

Some kinds of seizure disorders that start in childhood go away by adulthood. The most common form of childhood epilepsy, benign rolandic epilepsy, may not require any medical treatment at all (see the listing for rolandic epilepsy in this book's *Glossary* for more information).

Medical management of seizure disorders starts with a thorough evaluation from a pediatric or adult neurologist—an MD who specializes in the brain. Many medications are available to treat seizure disorders, some of which are better for specific types of seizures. It is important to have a thorough evaluation to try to define the seizure disorder as accurately as possible so that specific therapy can be started. Sometimes a person with epilepsy will need to try several different drugs to find the medication or combination of medications that works best and results in the least number of side effects. Some families try the ketogenic diet for children with seizure disorders to see if it decreases the number or intensity of the seizures.

If these methods do not control the seizures, and the seizures interfere with daily life, surgery may be recommended, particularly for temporal lobe epilepsy. There are several different surgical options available. Not all persons with epilepsy are candidates for surgery, but many people who do have surgery find that it greatly improves their lives.

The FDA has recently approved a device called the vagus nerve stimulator (VNS). It is surgically implanted in the chest and sends periodic mild electrical stimulation along the vagus nerve. In some cases, it decreases or eliminates seizures with minimal side effects.

The details of these and other epilepsy treatment methods are discussed in Chapter 5, *Medical Interventions*, and Chapter 6, *Other Interventions*.

Communication within the brain

Brain cells (neurons) are tiny ball-shaped cells with long arms called dendrites. There are actually several different types of neurons, each with a specific structure and purpose. Neurons communicate with each other through a complex interaction involving electrical impulses and chemical messengers known as neurotransmitters.

Neurotransmitters can only carry their messages to the right kind of neuron. They travel in the space between two neurons, searching for a receptor site where they can attach (bind) themselves. If a neurotransmitter molecule finds a place to attach itself, an electrical signal is generated within the neuron. Millions of these complicated neuron-to-neurotransmitter-to-neuron chain reactions may occur in a millisecond—so quickly that the time between perception and reaction seems instantaneous.

Neurotransmitters are active mostly in the central nervous system, but they have jobs to do throughout the body. For example, neurotransmitter receptor sites are also found in the digestive system, and some neurotransmitters are produced there as well as in the brain. That may be why so many people with seizures or migraine experience strange stomach sensations as part of their symptoms.

Some neurotransmitters are amino acids or proteins, while others are similar to the chemicals known as hormones. Hormones are secreted by the endocrine glands, which in turn are controlled by the brain. Hormonal changes can affect emotions. Some women with seizure disorders have a frequency pattern that is closely related to the hormone-driven menstrual cycle, and it's possible that other hormonal cycles also have an effect on seizure disorders.

Not enough is known about how the neurotransmitter system and the endocrine system interact, but among researchers seeking knowledge about seizure disorders, it is an area of great interest. What has been learned so far has already led to new treatments for epilepsy and provided information about why some drugs that reduce seizures also cause difficult physical side effects.

Kindling: A theory in progress

In a person with a seizure disorder, neurons within the seizure focus have a tendency toward electrical misfires. Most of the time their random "surges" cause no noticeable problems. Neighboring neurons ignore the misfires and continue on with their work as usual. But if the conditions are just right, a misfire may start a chain reaction, affecting nearby neurons that then spread the error to their neighbors, and so on.

Some researchers suspect that every time a seizure occurs, the brain becomes more disposed toward having seizures. This process, known as kindling, has so far been seen only in experiments using lab animals whose seizures were provoked with electrical or chemical stimulation. In lab animals, kindling occurs when a neuronal "spark" sets off the nervous system's version of a larger blaze: a seizure. Although the kindling process has not yet been documented in humans, the very latest research demonstrates the detrimental long-term effects of uncontrolled seizures, including worsening of seizure activity.[1] However, even if there is a human version of the kindling process, it is definitely different from the kindling process in lab animals—for example, doctors already know that even repeated use of electroconvulsive ("shock") therapy to treat psychiatric disorders does not cause epilepsy, even though it does provoke a controlled seizure.

Kindling is the focus of intense research right now, and more about how it works is being discovered every day. Hopefully this research will lead to better understanding of how epilepsy develops in humans. It may also lead to the development of better preventive medications for seizure disorders, with fewer side effects and risks than today's treatments.

There are many ideas about how a human kindling process might work. One theory is that the brain learns through repetition, so just as repeated exposure to the alphabet usually results in memorization, repeated seizures may make neural pathways "learn" to permit seizure activity. Another theory is that each seizure episode causes damage to neurons and neural pathways.

Even though neurologists don't fully understand kindling, they know enough to recommend that people with partial seizures take anti-epileptic drugs, even though their episodes might not look or sound as serious as tonic-clonic seizures. The medication is seen as a precautionary measure, as well as a treatment for any current distress.

Auras: A type of simple partial seizure

An aura, also known as a prodrome or the prodromal phase of a seizure, is actually a simple partial seizure. For many decades, seizure specialists talked about auras as if they were no more than some sort of epileptic early-warning system. It's true that many patients who have tonic-clonic seizures do have auras beforehand, although some do not. However, an aura is more than just a premonitory sensation.

Auras are highly individualized. Some people see flashing lights, others smell a strange odor, and some simply have an odd mental sensation, such as a floating feeling. It all depends on where the seizure focus is in the person's brain, and where the process catches hold.

Auras reported by people with seizure disorders may include the following:

- A sense of déjà vu: the feeling of having been somewhere before, when one has not
- A sense of jamais vu: the feeling that a familiar place is suddenly strange and unfamiliar
- Ringing or buzzing in the ears
- Hearing other sounds that are not there, ranging from bells to a clamor of human voices
- Smelling odors that are not there, including such pungent smells as gasoline, burning rubber, feces, peanuts, bananas, or even the scent of a specific perfume
- Feeling disoriented
- Feeling larger or smaller than normal, like Alice in Wonderland in her "drink me" phase

- Experiencing other distortions of perception, like feeling that the room is tilting or revolving
- Experiencing sudden dilation of pupils
- Feeling lightheaded
- Feeling dizzy
- Suffering from numbness in a part of the body
- Experiencing tremors in hands, feet, arms, or legs
- Feeling a spreading warmth or chilliness
- Feeling as though the stomach is rising, heaving, or being "pulled" upwards in the abdomen
- Feeling prickly sensations ("pins and needles"), especially on the feet and hands
- Feeling sudden emotions, such as dread, fear, anger, rage, happiness, or euphoria, that come "out of the blue" and are not related to the situation
- Seeing patterns or colors
- Suffering from sudden headaches, stomachaches, or other sorts of unpleasant or unusual physical sensations

While the aura is occurring, the person retains consciousness and may be able to continue having a conversation, driving, or working, although some types of auras are so distracting that it's hard to continue normal activity. An aura may be followed by a more recognizable complex partial, absence, or tonic-clonic seizure, although it may not occur right away.

Kindling and auras in other disorders

The terms kindling and aura are also sometimes used to describe similar phenomena experienced by some people with bipolar disorders (manic depression) and/or migraine attacks. The relationship between these conditions and seizure disorders is not thoroughly understood, although it appears that people with any form of epilepsy are also more likely to have a bipolar disorder or migraine than people who do not, and vice versa.

That said, the phenomena labeled as kindling and auras in bipolar disorders and migraine are significantly different from what people with epilepsy experience, and are different from each other as well. They may be related processes, but they are not identical.

Seizure phases

Doctors often use the terms pre-ictal, peri-ictal, ictal, inter-ictal, and post-ictal when they talk about the seizure experience. Ictal means during the seizure event itself, so pre- and peri-ictal mean before a seizure, inter-ictal means between seizures, and post-ictal means after a seizure. For example, post-ictal confusion is a period of disordered thinking that may occur right after a seizure.

Prodromal is another word used to describe the period just before a seizure, especially if it features an aura.

The neurology of seizures

Every process in the human body involves the brain, from the simplest movement to the most complex emotion. Accordingly, seizures can disrupt any process in the human body, from triggering involuntary physical movement to causing a person to temporarily lose bladder control or perceive flashing lights. The effect of a seizure depends on the location of its focus, how and where the electrical misfiring spreads, and how long the seizure lasts. The patient's age and health can also make a difference in seizure length and severity.

One hundred years ago, when the study of seizure disorders was still new, the brain was considered quite mysterious. By observing what happened to patients who had suffered head trauma, doctors figured out that damage to certain areas of the brain seemed to cause specific types of problems. They used these observations, along with information about the structure of the brain gathered from autopsies, to start making a map of the brain.

At first these brain maps were very simple. The brain was divided up into lobes and structures that could be seen with the naked eye, and the general purposes of these areas were investigated. Many of the basic principles of brain anatomy were revealed in the early years of research, but much more has been learned since, especially now that researchers have powerful tools for examining brain cells and for taking pictures of activity patterns in the living brain.

Indeed, the brain-mapping process is by no means complete. Today doctors know a lot about what different parts of the brain do—for example, they know which parts of the brain control major muscle movements, such as those needed for walking, because it is known that people with specific types of brain injuries must learn to walk all over again. However, even the very best neurologists cannot pinpoint all of the multiple brain activities and relationships involved in even the simplest normal activity, such as blinking your eyes, much less complex activities like speaking or learning.

It is now clear that the brain is an exceedingly complicated organ, and that important functions like emotional regulation, communication, and learning involve multiple areas of the brain working together.

Brain basics

If partial seizures affect you or someone you care about, it's helpful to understand the basics of brain anatomy. You don't have to become an expert, but learning how the brain is organized and how it carries messages makes it easier to understand what doctors are talking about when they're discussing seizures, treatments, and related issues. This section takes a "big picture" approach. The brain is really fascinating, so you may not want to stop here. Appendix A, *Resources*, lists some resources for more in-depth information.

The brain is cushioned by watery fluid on all sides in the skull. It resembles a huge, fleshy, shelled walnut in shape. Like a walnut, it has two distinct but tightly connected halves. These are called the left and right cerebral hemispheres—and while they appear to be mirror images of each other, similar-looking parts of each hemisphere may do different things.

Like a walnut's exterior, the brain's surface folds in and out. These wrinkles increase the surface area of the brain, which is divided by especially deep grooves called fissures or sulci. The deepest of these, the longitudinal fissure, runs down the middle of the brain from front to back, dividing the left and right hemispheres.

The brain contains several major nerves, such as the optic nerves that connect it to the eyes. It has no pain receptors of its own. Blood vessels carry oxygen and nutrients to all parts of the brain, and channels called aqueducts allow fluid to move through some areas.

The hindbrain is located at the very back of the brain, atop the spinal cord. Its lowest segment is the medulla oblongata, which controls respiration, heart rate, and other very basic body functions. It also includes the cerebellum, which is essential for coordinating muscle movements and preserving one's sense of balance. It communicates with the rest of the brain via a structure called the pons. This narrower, longer part of the brain is also called the brain stem, because the much larger forebrain balances on top of it like the cap of a droopy-sided mushroom on a stem. The locations of these parts of the brain are shown in Figure 1-1.

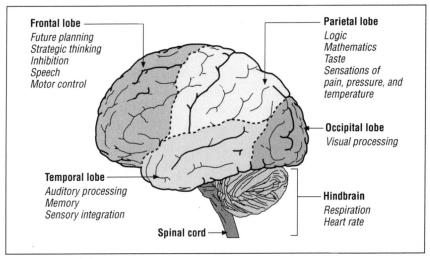

Figure 1-1. Basic brain anatomy

The forebrain, made up of the two cerebral hemispheres, consists of four major structures:

- **Frontal lobe.** The frontal lobe, located directly behind your forehead, is your mind's main planning center. It processes and stores information that helps you think ahead, use strategy, and respond to events based on past experiences and other knowledge. A small part of the frontal lobe aids in articulating speech, and another small strip of the frontal lobe helps control movement. Malfunctions in the frontal lobe may lead to poor planning, impulsiveness, and certain types of speech problems. Seizure activity in this lobe can cause temporary disorientation, loss of the ability to speak, or jerking limbs.

- **Parietal lobe.** The parietal lobe processes all sorts of sensory information from the body, including data about temperature, physical and atmospheric pressure, and pain. The parietal lobe is also involved in the sense of taste. When the parietal lobe is not functioning properly, sensory information may not process correctly, and the person may have a hard time making sense of his environment. During a seizure affecting the parietal lobe, strange physical sensations may be felt, such as a crushing pressure or a "tingle" in part of the body.

- **Occipital lobe.** The occipital lobe absorbs and processes visual information. Damage to this area is one cause of blindness from birth. Even people who are blind use the parietal lobe for some types of information processing. If this lobe is affected by a seizure, the person may "see" flashing lights or geometrical patterns before her eyes, or her vision may become blurred or distorted.

- **Temporal lobe.** The temporal lobe stores and retrieves memories and is involved in hearing. It is also believed to be the center where information taken in from the various senses is integrated, permitting complex thoughts, movements, and sensations to be formulated and acted upon. When temporal lobe activity is disrupted by seizures, the world becomes a confusing place. The brain has a hard time filtering out extra information, and sensory information and memories may start to blend together in unfamiliar ways. Sounds may be perceived as having colors, for example, or you may have an unsettling feeling of déja vu or jamais vu.

If you could look beyond the surface of the brain and inside these lobes, you would find a variety of other structures. One of the most important of these is the limbic lobe, also called the limbic system. Wrapped around the area where the forebrain and brain stem meet, the limbic lobe controls all sorts of very human impulses—sexuality, sensuality, emotions, and memory processing, just to name a few. Problems in the limbic system can cause loss of emotional intensity, heightened emotionality or impulsivity, impaired memory, and many other difficulties.

The part of the brain stem that the limbic lobe butts up against consists of several tiny but extraordinarily important structures: the thalamus, the hypothalamus, and the pineal gland. All sensory information passes through the thalamus before being sent to the forebrain for more advanced interpretation—except for information gathered via the sense of smell, which takes a different route.

The hypothalamus looks small, but it has a big role in managing everything from hunger to digestion to muscle contractions. It has direct control over the pituitary gland, which regulates the activities of most of the endocrine system, which in turn makes and uses hormones and similar chemicals.

The pineal gland's inner workings are still somewhat mysterious, but it is known to help govern the body's sense of time and rhythm, including regulation of the reproductive cycle. Malfunction in any of these areas can create distorted or blocked perceptions, severe digestive or hormonal problems, and other serious health problems.

Another important group of structures deep inside the brain are the tangles of specialized cells and tissue at the base of each hemisphere, known as the basal ganglia. The basal ganglia include the putamen, caudate nucleus, and amygdala. These structures control emotions (particularly panic and fear) and repetitive, automatic thoughts and muscle movements, and they ensure the smoothness of deliberate movements, among other functions. They are shown in Figure 1-2.

Conditions affecting the basal ganglia can result in fine or large tremors, tics, stereotypies (repetitive movements or postures), and difficulty in controlling repetitive thoughts and impulses, as is seen in obsessive-compulsive disorder and autism.

At the base of the medulla oblongata section of the hindbrain, the brain becomes the spinal cord, which is a long, tough bundle of nerve fibers that runs down the back and that is protected from harm by the vertebrae. The spinal cord and the brain are really a single oddly shaped organ, although most people tend to think of them as being separate. Together, they're called the central nervous system (CNS).

In fact, although this anatomy lesson has made much of the brain's different parts, it's important to remember that all of these areas are interconnected by a maze of nerve fibers, as well as the electrical and chemical message chains mentioned earlier in this chapter. What's more, the brain is an uncommonly adaptable organ, and can often route around damage in one area by giving another area new duties.

From the brain to the body

The brain and spinal cord communicate with the rest of the body via nerves, thin strings of tough fiber that extend throughout the body. The brain stem and spinal cord branch off into many nerves that carry information to and from every part of the body. Together, these nerves are known as the peripheral nervous system.

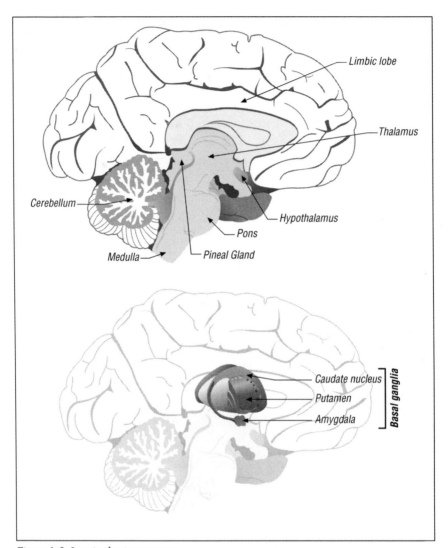

Figure 1-2. Interior brain structures

The peripheral nervous system carries commands from the central nervous system to various body parts and returns information gathered from your senses. For example, nerves close to the skin's surface are sensitive to touch, and tell the brain if they notice a crawling sensation. In response, your brain may trigger commands that cause you to absentmindedly brush a hand over the affected area, look at it, or scratch it.

Other nerves transmit information to and from the body's internal organs, including the heart, stomach, and intestines, as well as the sweat glands and the tiny muscles near the skin's surface whose contractions cause goose-bumps. These nerves, and the parts of the spinal cord and brain that control them, are called the visceral or autonomic nervous system.

Most of the time the workings of the peripheral, autonomic, and central nervous systems go completely unnoticed, because the majority of their interconnected activities concern basic physical functions: breathing, digesting food, producing hormones, pumping blood, and so on. Although it's possible to stop and purposefully make yourself aware of some of these processes (as during certain types of meditation that encourage control of breathing patterns or body temperature), most people pay no attention as long as everything is working well.

Seizure disorders constitute a disruption of the normal, smooth workings of these nervous systems as a whole. No matter where in the brain a person's seizure focus is located, it can have repercussions for many diverse physical and mental functions.

Seizure types and terms

Dozens of seizure types, seizure disorders, and medical conditions characterized by seizures have been identified. The *Glossary* lists many of these in alphabetical order. It also contains descriptive terms, synonyms, and alternative names, including a recap of many terms introduced earlier in this chapter.

What to do during a seizure

Partial seizures, whether simple or complex, rarely require special medical help during the event. If someone you are with is having a partial seizure that seems to be impairing his consciousness, the most important thing you can do is to simply keep him safe. Move dangerous objects out of his way, make sure he doesn't fall down, and wait with him until he regains full consciousness if possible. Do not try to restrain him. If he accidentally injures himself, seek appropriate medical help.

A very few people with partial seizures involving the temporal lobe or amygdala become aggressive or violent, either during or after a seizure. It is almost unheard of for a person with epilepsy to attack someone during or after a seizure, unless someone grabs or tries to restrain him, so just safeguard yourself and others who may be nearby, and seek help for the person who is having a seizure. Again, restraining him will probably just make the situation worse, as he cannot control this behavior.

If a partial seizure progresses to become a tonic-clonic seizure, the person may fall to the ground and have convulsions. As with a partial seizure, remove any dangerous objects from the area. You may also want to remove eyeglasses to prevent breakage, and loosen any tight clothing. There's no need to put anything in his mouth, and it might be dangerous for you to try. Don't worry—he can't swallow his tongue. If you can, turn the person onto his side to prevent him from swallowing saliva or vomit. Just let the seizure run its course.

There's no need for emergency help unless the person accidentally injures himself, stops breathing, or continues to have several tonic-clonic seizures, one after another. If he stops breathing, call for emergency help and then use mouth-to-mouth resuscitation until the ambulance comes.

After a tonic-clonic seizure, a person usually feels tired and disoriented. Stay with him until he feels well enough to go about his business.

If you have a seizure disorder yourself, it can be helpful to wear a medical alert bracelet in case you become disoriented or behave in other ways that might make people think you are drunk or on drugs. Some people who have partial seizures carry an information card in their wallet that can be given to concerned passersby or the police if necessary. Strategies for coping with seizures that occur in public are discussed in Chapter 3, *Living with Partial Seizure Disorders*.

CHAPTER 2

Diagnosis

THIS CHAPTER DISCUSSES choosing a qualified specialist and navigating the diagnostic process. It outlines the current diagnostic criteria for partial seizure disorders, and will help you understand the diagnostic tools and methods that you may encounter. This chapter also includes brief sections on other disorders that can contribute to or be mistaken for partial seizures, including attention deficit disorder, bipolar disorder, and migraine.

Getting a diagnosis

Most parents begin their search for help with their child's pediatrician, and most adults start by talking things over with their general practitioner. That's a good place to start, but while most primary care physicians are experts in strep throat, stomachaches, and other common medical problems, they need to refer their patients with complex medical problems to specialists.

Diagnosing partial seizure disorders can be quite difficult. Unless you have a recognizable seizure right in front of your doctor or during an EEG, diagnosis usually requires a lengthy process of observation, testing, and elimination. That can be quite a trial for patients, since it requires investigating various medical explanations (such as hypoglycemia or migraine), ruling out psychiatric conditions, and having tests for seizure activity done by a specialist. Patients sometimes endure a variety of intrusive examinations, or are even prescribed the wrong medications, while continuing to experience episodes of seizure activity.

Personal circumstances and secondary medical problems, such as psychiatric illness, sometimes cloud the picture even more. Almost twenty years passed between his first symptoms and a diagnosis for 33-year-old Larry:

> *Initially, I wasn't aware that there was anything physiologically wrong with me. My father was an alcoholic who unfortunately got excessively*

abusive when drinking. I don't normally speak about what happened throughout my childhood, but I think if you're aware of my background you'll understand why it took ages for a diagnosis to be made.

Once I had reached puberty, I noticed that there were occasions when I would have what I now know as "auras." Once I left home, however, things appeared to settle down. However, I know now that the rapid mood swings I experienced (I could go from total euphoria, to suicidal depression, to tears, to a blind rage in a matter of minutes) were all part of my epilepsy.

It was only after I got married that any investigations into my mood swings got started. My wife had to virtually threaten me with divorce before I would even accept that anything could possibly be wrong with me. Thank God she did. When I initially went in to speak to the doctor, he thought it might be clinical depression and started me on Prozac. This did absolutely nothing for me. He then started treating me for bipolar disorder. Let me tell you, lithium is not a fun drug to be on, and it didn't do anything for me either. I was then referred to a psychologist, as the doctor felt perhaps what had happened in the past might be what was causing these emotional mood swings. After six months of intensive therapy, I was informed that I was psychologically well-balanced and adjusted (gee, I could have told them that). I was then referred to a psychiatrist, who immediately sent me for an EEG. Once he got the results back, which definitely showed some "weird" electrical activity, I started on carbamazepine. This has proved to significantly reduce the mood swings. Now I see a neurologist also.

It's worth noting that carbamazepine is also used to treat bipolar disorder, which is probably the psychiatric disorder most often confused with partial seizures. It's often difficult, as in Larry's case, to tell one from the other, and it's certainly possible for the two to overlap. If your doctor isn't sure, he will probably rely on evidence from an EEG, as Larry's did.

If the EEG evidence is inconclusive, doctors may move on to brain imaging, order psychiatric tests, or even simply try different medications to see what works. It's hard to play this waiting game, especially if you are a parent worried about your child's well-being, or an adult coping with impairment that may affect your ability to drive, work, and live a normal life. You may wish fervently that your doctor would just prescribe something quickly. Unfortunately, the medications prescribed to treat seizure disorders are not to be taken lightly. Every single one of them has the potential for side effects, sometimes serious ones, if they are prescribed to patients who don't need them. Conscientious doctors want to be sure that they've left no stone unturned before these drugs are tried. If these medications are right for you, they are well worth the risk. If they are not, they could cause additional health problems.

This does not mean that you should be forced to wait for months, even years, while your primary care physician or HMO figures out what to do. Your best bet is to request an urgent referral for an expert evaluation. Most of the time, a board-certified neurologist with expertise in partial seizure disorders is the best person to perform an evaluation (see "Choosing a specialist," later in this chapter).

If you have additional concerns, such as developmental delay in a child or the presence of other health problems that have made diagnosis difficult in the past, you should probably seek a team of specialists who will work together (see "Multidisciplinary evaluations," later in this chapter).

Getting to a specialist

Unless you will be paying your doctors directly or have a health plan that allows you to seek the help of a specialist without a referral, you must put the diagnostic process in motion by requesting a consultation appointment with your child's pediatrician or your general practitioner. This kind of appointment is a little different from the typical "height check, weight check, immunization booster, your throat looks fine" visit. In fact, it may take place in a meeting room or office rather than in an examination room. It should also be longer in length: a half-hour at least, preferably an hour.

Accurate, detailed records are the most important thing you can contribute at this appointment. For children, these should include dates of the usual "baby book" milestones (first step, first word, etc.), as well as an account of what parents, teachers, or other caregivers have observed during the episodes that you suspect may be seizures. For older children and adults, the doctor will ask for a thorough description of these episodes from the patient, although the perspective of a spouse or friend is also valuable.

Your doctor may ask for a lot of details about your family's health history, including medical problems, mental health issues, and whether anyone else in the family has a seizure disorder. These questions may seem intrusive, but they are important.

Before the consultation appointment, take the time to ask older relatives what they know. Often people with partial seizure disorders were never officially diagnosed. You may hear tales of a grandparent's strange episodes, or secret trips to the hospital. On the other hand, some people are still very reluctant to talk about epilepsy or symptoms that they feel might indicate a mental illness. You may need to go so far as sleuthing through medical records or diaries in the attic, or questioning doctors who knew older family members. Physicians are duty-bound not to give you personal information about living persons, but they may be more forthcoming about patients who are deceased. Once you have this family history in hand, you might want to put it in very simple "family tree" form for your physician.

Keeping a daily diary is also an excellent way to prepare for the consultation appointment (see Appendix B, *Seizure Diary*). Many families and patients learn a great deal during this process. Use your diary to record activities, diet, and behaviors each day for a period of two weeks or more, with the time and duration of activities, behaviors, and "episodes" noted. Not only can this diary provide a very complete picture of the person to a professional, it can also help to identify patterns. If you can, use a calendar, personal diaries, medical notes, and your own recollections to create a rough chart of any episodes of unusual behavior or sensation over the past year or so. That can help a doctor identify possible triggers of seizure-like behavior, such as stress or the use of a particular medication.

If you can, catch one or more episodes on videotape. Video is an excellent tool for helping your doctor understand the problem. You may be able to rent or borrow a video camera if you don't own one.

If you or your child has seen other doctors, you must sign releases to have these medical records transferred to the primary care physician before the consultation appointment. Helpful school records can also be transferred if a signed release is on file. Transfers always seem to take longer than you would expect, so get releases taken care of early, and make sure the records were actually sent and received. Alternatively, if you have your own copies of these records (and you should), you may photocopy them and deliver them to the doctor yourself.

You should also summarize your concerns in writing. The records already mentioned can help you gather your thoughts. You don't have to be an eloquent writer to express what worries you. If you prefer, you can jot down a simple list of concerns or questions rather than writing whole paragraphs. Some people send this summary of concerns to the doctor in advance, while others prefer to use it as an agenda for discussion during the consultation.

You might also want to talk to a nurse or physician's assistant who works closely with your doctor. In large medical practices and HMOs, nurses and assistants are an important part of the organization. They can be allies for people who need referrals to specialists or even just a listening ear. If you are lucky enough to find a knowledgeable and sympathetic nurse, her input can help greatly.

If possible, your information and the complete medical file should be available to the doctor at least a week before the consultation appointment. These should be accompanied by a request that she read the material in advance and review the patient's file before the meeting. You want to ensure that your case is fresh in your doctor's mind at the consultation appointment.

When you arrive for the consultation, bring any additional records you have gathered, copies of your earlier letter (just in case it never reached the doctor), your summary of concerns, and a prioritized list of any questions that you want to ask. You can bring a small notebook or tape recorder as well, so you can keep a record of the discussion.

At the consultation, your general practitioner will simply listen, discuss your difficulties, and recommend the next course of action. Some will use a set of standard questions about behavior, development, or symptoms to screen you or your child.

Checklists and guidelines are great, but there's really no substitute for knowledge and experience. If your doctor is reluctant to refer you to a specialist, there are several responses you can make:

- Go back over your evidence, explaining how these episodes are affecting you or your child at school, at home, and in the community.

- Let the doctor know what interventions you've already tried, such as treatment for other disorders, counseling, or lifestyle changes.

- Emphasize any special factors that you feel support the possibility that you or your child could have a partial seizure disorder. These include knowledge that other people in your family have been diagnosed with a seizure disorder; presence in your family of other disorders with strong links to seizure disorders, such as bipolar disorders or migraine; and suggestions by a previous doctor or other professional (teacher, social worker, etc.) that you or your child should be evaluated for a seizure disorder.

- Ask the doctor to put his refusal to refer in writing. This may not be something he'd like to commit to paper, so you might end up getting the referral after all.

- If the doctor does put his refusal in writing, you can choose to call your diagnostic facility of choice and set up an appointment directly. Be prepared to pay for this visit out-of-pocket. However, if the specialists confirm your suspicions, you should be able to bill your insurance company for reimbursement due to refusal of an appropriate referral.

- If the doctor won't refer and won't put his refusal in writing, you can still "self-refer," but it will be harder to get reimbursed. You should send a letter to your primary care physician explaining why you have made this choice over his objections. Send a copy to your HMO and insurance company as well. This creates a paper record, allowing you to pursue a claim for improper refusal later on, if warranted.

- Go up the chain of command if your doctor is in a managed care organization or HMO. In these medical groups there is a board that considers patient complaints. You can petition the board to approve your referral even if the primary care provider refuses. Usually this is done in writing, not in person.

- Talk to a special needs coordinator at your HMO. Many HMOs now have these coordinators to ensure that patients with disabilities or chronic health conditions have their needs met. The special needs coordinator can often suggest creative work-arounds or tell you who to talk to. Many are empowered to act as a temporary case manager to help patients who are still in the diagnostic stage.

In the US, most doctors share the risks and expenses of caring for special-needs patients (including specialist referrals) with business partners or an HMO group. Doctors who make too many referrals can face financial penalties, even if the extra services were absolutely necessary. Physicians may also feel constrained by directives from insurance companies, which want to minimize expenses.

Iain feels that he waited too long for his doctor to make a specialist referral:

> Certainly I've had more trouble getting diagnosed with epilepsy than for more physical ailments. I went to my general practitioner and presented classic (as I found out later) temporal lobe epilepsy symptoms, and even after I'd gone back several times it was still put down to being an "adolescent thing." It wasn't until I had a grand mal at age 18 that I was actually diagnosed, but that wasted five years of potential treatment time.

Low-income Americans who are uninsured face the biggest barrier of all: lack of access to healthcare. Your county health or mental health department should be your first stop. Your school district may also provide some diagnostic and therapeutic assistance in areas related to classroom behavior and performance. There are special medical programs and facilities available for low-income families and for children with handicapping conditions, although they often have long waiting lists. Chapter 7, *Healthcare and Insurance*, provides many ideas for getting diagnostic help and ongoing care if you or your child is not covered by private insurance.

In Canada and Europe, where the single-payer system of nationalized healthcare predominates, doctors have a different set of constraints on their ability to make referrals. Resources are focused on providing basic healthcare to everyone, so there are fewer specialists than in the US. Parents who want prompt care for their children may be forced to pay out-of-pocket to doctors who practice outside the national healthcare scheme. The expenses can be considerable. Some families have been able to gain faster access to specialists with help from a sympathetic social worker or health visitor, or have called on advocacy groups for assistance.

In countries where neither private insurance nor the single-payer model predominates, parents should seek out—and pay for—a specialist directly, without going through a preliminary consultation appointment. Reduced-fee or free help may be available through state-run hospitals and clinics, medical facilities owned by religious orders or charities, or individual physicians who are willing to take a case at a lower cost than usual.

No matter what kind of healthcare system you face, it pays to be persistent. Barb, age 43, was diagnosed thirteen years ago as having partial seizures:

> I had been having frequent feelings that "I've done this before," "I've seen this before," many déja vu feelings. I decided to see a doctor to check into this. Mind you, I had no idea that a seizure problem could be there.

After explaining all of my feelings to this professional, I was told that I was imagining things and that I needed to see a psychiatrist. I've done some crazy things in my life, but I didn't feel that I was imagining this.

A good friend of my mother's was the president of our state's epilepsy association at the time. During a phone conversation, my mom mentioned what I went to a doctor for and the reaction of this MD. The friend told my mother that I was having seizures and to get me to a neurologist soon. And that was that.

Choosing a specialist

Depending on how your quest for an evaluation goes, your doctor may suggest that your first appointment be with a neurologist, a psychiatrist, a psychologist, or a team of specialists working together.

As a specialist in brain disorders, a neurologist will usually be your primary source for diagnostic help and continuing care, including prescriptions. If you have other professionals, such as a general practitioner or a psychiatrist, involved in your healthcare, he may ask them to administer tests (psychiatric tests or blood tests, for example), and he may direct their treatment choices later on. For that reason, it's important to find a board-certified neurologist who specializes in seizure disorders and who is up to date on the latest research about partial seizure disorders in particular.

You might begin your search for a specialist by calling one of the support or advocacy groups listed in Appendix A, *Resources*, such as the Epilepsy Foundation of America.

Neurologists who are epilepsy specialists may call themselves epileptologists. Epileptologists are usually associated with a special epilepsy clinic or hospital-based program. The National Association of Epilepsy Centers is an organization of such facilities (see Appendix A for additional contact information).

Most epileptologists will see patients with any type of seizure disorders, although a few specialize in a specific form or forms of epilepsy, or work primarily with children, brain-injured patients who have seizures, or another specific group.

Internet discussion groups like EPILEPSY-L can also be a good source of tips and advice about doctors in your area. The value of support groups, both traditional and online, is discussed in Chapter 3, *Living with Partial Seizure Disorders*. The best time to make first contact with these groups is when you are still in search of a diagnosis and help. You can avoid dead ends, unqualified doctors, and much heartache by tapping into these resources right away. Even if it turns out that the problems are due to another condition, you'll be glad to have found out so quickly.

Iain called on family members for help in finding a new neurologist:

> *My first neurologist tried me on phenytoin, which worked for a bit, and then phenytoin and Tegretol, but when that didn't work he told me that there was nothing that could be done. I decided to find a new neuro! I guess I'm lucky in that the rest of my family is in the medical profession, so I made use of their contacts to find someone. I shudder to think what would have happened without those contacts.*

Another source for referrals is the neurology department of a nearby medical school. Many medical schools have excellent clinics staffed by both experienced doctors and residents who are learning the ropes. Some of the foremost experts in partial seizure disorders are affiliated with university programs. These doctors are often (but not always!) aware of the latest research findings and treatments.

Two important indicators of expertise are board certification and a working relationship with a good hospital, preferably one affiliated with a university medical school. Board-certified means that the doctor has completed an extensive training program, has already practiced in her specialty for some years, and meets the most rigorous qualifications in the field as set by the American Board of Psychiatry and Neurology, an official board of her peers. You can reach the board at (847) 945-7900. You can also check a doctor's certification status with the American Board of Medical Specialties at (800) 776-CERT or on the Web at *http://www.certifieddoctor.org*.

Once you have identified a neurologist you would like to work with, call her office to make sure she is currently taking new patients. Ask specifically if she sees patients with partial seizure disorders and, if you are a parent, if she sees patients your child's age. You may also want to ask if she has worked with your health plan or HMO before. Insurance regulations, or the rules of your national health plan, usually govern just how you go about accessing a specialist. Problems that frequently occur, and ideas for dealing with them, are covered in Chapter 7.

Multidisciplinary evaluations

A multidisciplinary evaluation is a team approach to diagnosis, and it is usually the best way to help patients who have symptoms that could be caused by two or more different conditions, or who have multiple medical problems.

For partial seizure disorder evaluations, the multidisciplinary team should include your general practitioner, who has the best knowledge of your general health; a neurologist with expertise in partial seizure disorders; and one or more other specialists: experts in migraine or genetic disorders, a developmental pediatrician, a psychiatrist, or a psychologist, for example.

Physicians of all stripes collaborate to help patients, but it's still fairly rare for them to work together directly by seeing the patient at the same time. Usually each specialist will see you individually, and then consult about your case at a meeting, in a written report, or over the phone. Sometimes the patient or her family will handle coordination between team members, but sometimes the services of a professional case manager may be required. Case management services can be provided through a clinic or hospital, a social services agency, or a private health advocate.

Gia, mother of 5-year-old James, says:

> Our introduction to pediatric neurologists began with the multidisciplinary team at a major children's hospital that followed our son during his hospitalization for brain surgery, so our first experience was with a pediatric neurologist located about two hours away from our home. Although this connection with a leading hospital had its advantages, there were distinct disadvantages: our son had his one and only moderately severe tonic-clonic seizure in the middle of the night, and it required overnight hospitalization. Since he had been treated only by the specialists two hours away, no one knew him at our local facility. We learned the hard way that we needed to select a local pediatric neurologist to oversee seizure management. After that episode, we've made regular office visits and phone calls to our local pediatric neurologist, and we visit and update our specialists at the children's hospital as needed.

Psychiatrists and psychologists

A psychiatrist or psychologist can be an important part of a multidisciplinary team for diagnosing partial seizure disorders. These professionals specialize in treating the behavioral and social aspects of all disorders, not just mental illness. They can help you learn coping strategies for dealing with your symptoms. In addition, these professionals can assist your neurologist by administering tests of brain function.

Although most people with partial seizure disorders do not have psychological problems, some do see a psychologist or psychiatrist for treatment of other conditions, or for help with psychological issues related to partial seizure disorders. In addition, if you have a health plan that limits your ability to access a neurologist for medication management, a psychiatrist might handle your medication.

Many people don't have a clear understanding of what psychiatrists and psychologists do. There's a common belief that they help people cope with problems brought on by bad experiences, but that's only partly true. Most of what these professionals do is treating biological illnesses that affect the brain. Both practitioners can offer emotional support and teach practical coping strategies, but psychiatrists, who are medical doctors, can also prescribe drugs.

Iain says a psychologist might have been a good addition to his treatment team:

> I've never worked with either a psychiatrist or a psychologist in this context. I wish something like this had been offered. I get the feeling that the whole epilepsy thing knocked a massive hole in my already shaky adolescent confidence. And it has affected me a lot since—life has been a battle to get my confidence back. More assistance from the beginning to help me come to terms with the epilepsy and stuff would have been great.

To ensure communication and teamwork, your choice of psychiatrists or psychologists will probably be limited to doctors your neurologist already has a working relationship with. As with evaluating a neurologist, your main criteria will be knowledge of partial seizure disorders, whether others have recommended the practitioner, and board certification.

When you see a psychiatrist or psychologist, your visit is unlikely to resemble the stereotypical trip to the shrink as seen in a Woody Allen film. Most eschew those funny-looking chaise lounges these days, so you're more likely to find an office furnished with a desk, chairs, overfilled bookshelves, and perhaps some toys.

Psychiatrists and psychologists who work with children usually talk to the parents first, with or without the child present. Then they spend some time with the child alone, and finally chat with both parents and child. They may administer standardized tests, or you may simply converse about your concerns.

When working with adult patients, psychiatrists and psychologists may combine discussion with formal testing in one or more appointments.

Pay attention to your feelings in this first meeting, because the best indicator for success in working with a psychiatrist or psychologist is your rapport. The core of your treatment with this professional will be open communication and trust. Sometimes a particular doctor is not a good fit for you or your child.

Regardless of her personal style, a psychiatrist or psychologist should always be a good listener. She should be willing to answer questions, whether an adult patient, a child, or a child's parents ask them.

The psychiatrist or psychologist may see you only once, she may see you on an occasional basis for medication management, or in a few cases she may see you for weekly or more frequent therapy sessions. You, however, must live with your symptoms or your child's challenges every day of the year, in all sorts of situations. A conscientious practitioner knows that your observations and input are essential at every stage of diagnosis and treatment, and considers you a collaborator in your own treatment.

Darrell, father of Reese, says:

> I'm definitely one of those parents who went into major terror mode after my son's first tonic-clonic seizure. In fact, I'm still working my way out of that, two years of therapy later.
>
> The thing to remember is that as parents of people with epilepsy, we also have a unique perspective on the illness. With a young child, it's really not possible to say that only the child has the illness. Epilepsy is a family medical issue, in my opinion, especially uncontrolled epilepsy. Everyone has to be aware of it, educated about it, and prepared to offer the appropriate first aid if need be. When your seven-year-old starts having seizures, it's simply impossible as a parent not to try to take their fear and suffering on for them, even though you rationally know that you cannot. I can remember praying to God almighty to give me the epilepsy and

spare Reese, and that's not some kind of martyr syndrome. I honestly believed that it would have been better that way.

In any event, it seems to be very common for a child's seizures to affect the whole family, hence the Epilepsy Foundation of America's recommendation that family counseling be a standard part of treatment for epilepsy. I wholeheartedly agree. It's been the only thing that saved my relationship with my son, I can tell you.

Other team members

In some health plans, a therapist, counselor, or specialized social worker acts as a gatekeeper for mental health services: you must see this person before you are allowed to see a psychiatrist. Therapists, counselors, and social workers can also administer many of the standardized tests used in the diagnostic process, observe patients and take notes, and talk to patients and parents about family, medical, social, and educational history. They can also support the diagnostic team by finding out what kind of information and support the patient and his family need during the diagnostic process. After the diagnosis has been made, they can provide more information, offer therapy sessions, help families locate resources in the community, and provide a listening ear when needed.

Your regular MD is also an important part of the team and should be kept informed. After all, you will probably see your MD more frequently than you see a specialist, and many health conditions can affect your seizure disorder if not properly treated.

Finally, if you see a specialist for treatment of a health condition that could impact your seizures, such as diabetes or hormonal problems, this doctor should be part of your treatment team as well.

Diagnostic tests

Your very first appointment after your initial consultation with your primary care physician will probably concentrate on intake procedures—and that means paperwork with a capital "P." If you will be getting a diagnosis through a special clinic or an epilepsy program at a hospital, and perhaps receiving ongoing services thereafter, there will be many forms for you to fill out before you finally get a chance to see a doctor. These will probably include billing and insurance forms, waivers that permit the doctor to get your medical records from other places, and sometimes a medical history or checklist.

At some clinics that specialize in epilepsy, the intake process also includes interviewing the patient and/or parents. This interview may be conducted by a social worker. The histories you prepared for your earlier primary care provider consultation will make this go much more smoothly.

During the intake process, you'll be asked many questions. One that you should ask is who will be in charge of coordinating practitioners and services as you move through the diagnostic process and into treatment. This person can be your primary contact and help you be prepared for each step along the way.

Meeting your neurologist

Neurologists usually work in a regular-looking medical office, complete with exam table and scales. The neurologist will begin your first appointment by taking a brief medical history and asking any questions that your file brought to mind (in some cases an assistant will do this before you see the neurologist). Then he'll move on to discussing the symptoms that have brought you to his office.

The first tests he'll administer are a set of deceptively simple exercises that, when observed by an expert, offer many clues about brain function and possible areas of concern. He may ask you to do things like touch your finger to your nose, stand on one foot, or stand with your eyes closed.

Indeed, the most important diagnostic device a neurologist can possess is an expert power of observation. If you have the right person on your team, he has seen many patients with many types of nervous-system problems. He keeps up with the latest reports from medical journals, and he delights in learning more about the frontiers of this medical field. When you or your child are in his office, he will watch movements, speech patterns, and ways of thinking to see what clues they offer about brain function. Don't let that intimidate you—it's exactly what you've come to a specialist for.

If you prepared symptom diaries, family or developmental histories, or videotapes for your general practitioner, make sure your neurologist also gets copies of these. Videotapes can be especially helpful, since it's fairly unlikely that you will experience a seizure while in your neurologist's office.

Ron offers his philosophy about choosing and working with neurologists:

> *For years and years I had been seeing a general neurologist. This past summer I switched to a doctor at a neurologic clinic in a hospital. He's an epileptologist, and only treats patients with epilepsy. It really makes a big difference to see one of these doctors. They know the medications better, and have a much better understanding of different seizures.*
>
> *A patient should be prepared to answer a lot of questions. Some of these are difficult to answer. The doctor will probably ask something like, "How does it feel when you have these partial seizures?" If you go to a doctor because you have an earache, chances are pretty good that doctor may have had an earache at some point in his or her life. Or if you have a broken bone, the doctor can see that. But partial seizures usually cannot be seen, as opposed to grand mals. So I would suggest that patients give some thought as to how to answer this question before they get to the doctor's office. For instance, I have come up with this explanation: "My partial seizures feel very much the way you feel when you have a high temperature." I discovered this when I had come down with a bad case of the flu and had a very high temperature. Only I didn't know I had the flu, I thought I was having partial seizures. An explanation like this can help the doctor decide what type of epilepsy one has, and how to treat it.*

Don't be shy about asking to see the results of any diagnostic tests your neurologist or other members of the team use. If you don't understand what a test measures, how it is scored, or what the results mean, ask questions until you're satisfied.

Electroencephalograms

Once the basic neurological exam is out of the way, your neurologist will move on to using some high-tech tools. The most widely used device for diagnosing any type of seizure disorder is the electroencephalograph, or EEG. This machine measures the electrical activity generated by the brain. There is no health risk from an EEG, with the exception of special types called depth or subdural grid EEGs (see the list items "Depth EEG", and "Subdural grid EEG" later in this chapter) that are rarely used unless a patient is being evaluated for brain surgery.

To prepare for an EEG, wash your hair before the test and avoid conditioner, creams, hairspray, oil, gels, and elaborate hairstyles. Sometimes small children and people with behavior disorders may be given a mild sedative before an EEG is done. You should avoid caffeinated drinks for a day before the test.

For the most common type of EEG test, usually called a scalp EEG, the neurologist or an EEG technician sticks 21 or 22 electrodes to the scalp with gooey glue. Each little disk is strategically placed to capture the brain wave activity from a different region of the brain, and each is attached to a wire called a lead. You may feel a bit like Frankenstein's monster while all the electrodes and leads are attached, but you won't feel any pain. Because the heart's electrical activity can skew EEG results, it is usually monitored by a separate electrode on the chest.

The loose end of each lead is attached to the EEG machine itself, which amplifies the tiny amount of activity to make graphing it possible. Depending on which kind of output device is being used, the EEG machine represents your brain's electrical output as patterns on a piece of paper, on a computer screen, or both. Each electrode's report is graphed as a line in a document or screen display called an electroencephalogram. As brain activity occurs, the voltage changes, and so does the shape of these lines.

The basic type of EEG test lasts between half an hour and two hours. During that time, the neurologist or an assistant may try some things that could provoke a seizure. You might be asked to look at a flashing light (photic stimulation) or breathe rapidly for several minutes (hyperventilate).

If you catch a glimpse of your brain waves on the printout or computer monitor, don't be alarmed if you see odd patterns and scribbles. Every time one of your muscles moves, a corresponding blip will appear on the EEG. These normal changes in electrical activity are called muscle or movement artifacts. Movement of the electrodes also generates what EEG technicians call electrode pops. If the EEG is being done in the emergency room while the patient is hooked up to an IV, a spike may appear each time a drip of saline solution is released. Finally, normal brain activity can also produce spiky patterns that could be misinterpreted as seizures by someone who isn't familiar with the wide variety of normal patterns.

Indeed, reading EEG results takes careful training and a great deal of practice. The reader must filter out all of the meaningless patterns to see if anything unusual emerges. Seizures appear as changes in activity—spikes, waves, or other pattern shifts—but only an expert like a neurologist can tell these from artifacts, electrode pops, and heart activity.

Any abnormal spikes or waves seen during the EEG may be limited to certain parts of the brain (focal) or they may spread to many parts of the brain (generalized). If you have a partial seizure disorder, any disturbance may start out as focal, although it can spread to other parts of the brain later. Some types of seizures produce very distinctive patterns.

If seizure activity is detected, the neurologist may begin discussing treatment with you right away, or you may be scheduled for further testing to help him collect more detailed information about your seizures.

Some people have abnormal brain activity all the time. This can be a sign of low-level seizures occurring very frequently, or an indicator of other types of brain-based problems. If you fall into this group, your neurologist will probably move directly to trying one of the brain imaging techniques discussed later in this chapter.

On the other hand, your first EEG could look basically normal. This doesn't mean you don't have epilepsy; it means you did not have a seizure during the EEG, and you do not have grossly abnormal brain waves at all times. Studies have shown that standard, 20- to 30-minute EEG tests show no seizure activity in 40 and 50 percent of cases in which the patient is definitely diagnosed with epilepsy at a later date.[1] Indeed, it's fairly rare for someone to have a seizure during an EEG. More frequently, what catches the neurologist's attention are brief patterns, lasting for one second or less, of unusual activity. These almost imperceptible changes are called inter-ictal or epileptiform discharges. They occur between seizures in people with epilepsy, and there are many different types of them. Most of the time, it's observation of these inter-ictal discharges that allows a firm diagnosis of epilepsy to be made, especially in people with partial seizures.

If there are still good reasons to believe that a patient has a seizure disorder despite a negative first EEG, the neurologist will order a follow-up EEG. This test may be just like the first one, or it may be set up to increase the likelihood of seeing seizure activity during the test by trying one of the following EEG types:

- Sleep-deprived EEG. This type of EEG is administered after a period of sleep deprivation. Sleep deprivation lowers the seizure threshold dramatically, and some kinds of seizures are more likely to occur in deep sleep. For this test, the patient must stay up all or most of the night and then come in for a scalp EEG in the morning. Once the electrodes are hooked up and the neurologist has had an initial look at brain activity, you can fall into the deep sleep that you've been craving for hours. The dual challenge of sleep deprivation and deep sleep often evokes seizure activity.

Keeping kids awake is a special challenge. Lucy, mother of 10-year-old Harry, tells how her family handled it:

My husband took the early shift, playing board games and watching movies until about 1 a.m. Then I got up (after four hours of sleep!), made popcorn, and we watched a movie of Harry's choice. After the movie, we went to the International House of Pancakes for a 3 a.m. breakfast. In the car we sang silly songs. We got back to the house, played some more board games and cards, then at about 5 a.m. went to a 24-hour Wal-Mart. Harry spent a lot of time there studying the fishing lures and baits, plus of course the toy section. From there, the first light of morning was just beginning to show, so we headed to a playground! Then we went back home.

Wouldn't you know it, he then proceeded to have a seizure at the house! I loaded him in the car and took him on to the hospital. The hardest part was keeping him awake after the seizure. For the thirty-minute drive to the hospital, I had the windows down and rock music blaring on the radio. I poked him at every stoplight to keep him semi-awake.

We did get the sleep-deprived EEG done. He was awake the first few minutes, then fell asleep on the table. That is what they want, so they get both the waking and sleeping states. He absolutely refused to cooperate with the strobe light, and we finally gave up on that part.

- **EEG with special leads.** In these types of EEGs, the neurologist obtains more information by adding additional leads. One goes up the nose and into the throat area behind it (the nasopharynx). Another can be attached near the base of the neck. A third type is a sphenoidal lead, which is inserted on the side of the face about one inch in front of the ear.

- **Ambulatory EEG.** Portable EEG machines are sometimes used to monitor a patient non-stop for one or more days. Some EEG machines are less portable than others, and work best when the patient is already in the hospital and not very active. Others are small and light enough to permit the monitor to go home with you. When you're having an ambulatory EEG done, your main role is to make sure you stay hooked up, and to take careful notes about any unusual sensations or behaviors you have. The doctor can then look at the EEG record and see if there was abnormal electrical discharge during those events. You'll need instructions on how to keep the electrodes and leads connected, how to operate the machine, and what activities to avoid while being monitored. Make sure you feel comfortable with handling any problems that could occur before you go home with the monitor. If your doctor orders a 24-hour EEG or talks about EEG telemetry, this is what she means.

Five-year-old James had this type of EEG at a very early age, explains his mother, Gia:

> *James had a five-day EEG when he was 3 years old. It was especially hard for him because he is extremely sensitive to smells. The ether-based glue they used to attach leads to the head was so overwhelming he just screamed the whole time. The wires were long enough to let him get out of bed and move around the room and doorway. There were several kids having this test, so they were able to meet just outside their rooms. They played games, made play dough sculptures, and they heard a lot of stories.*

- **Videotaped EEG.** This type of EEG is done while the patient is also being videotaped. By comparing the patient's visible and self-reported symptoms with the EEG data, subtle correlations may be found.

- **BEAM EEG.** Brain Electrical Activity Monitoring, or BEAM, is a computerized EEG technique that uses extra electrode channels to detect and eliminate artifacts. It employs lights and sounds to elicit seizure activity, lasts longer than a typical EEG, and compares results against a database of information on seizures in patients matched for age and gender. BEAM testing requires very specialized interpretation skills and remains controversial among epileptologists, many of whom feel it is misused in some clinical settings.

- **Depth EEG.** This type of EEG requires implanting electrodes temporarily into the brain. Obviously, the head must be absolutely still during this procedure. Your head will be placed in a frame that is pinned to your skull. CT or MRI scanning will then help the doctor decide where the electrodes should be placed. With great care and precision, the neurosurgeon drills through the skull and inserts flexible electrodes into those parts of the brain where seizure activity is suspected. There are no nerve endings inside the skull, so this will cause you no pain, but some people experience discomfort despite the use of local anesthesia. After the operation you'll probably have a nasty headache. Your head will be wrapped in a bandage, and your scalp will be sore. It will take about a month to heal after the procedure is done. Depth electrodes, also called subdural electrodes, are generally not used in those areas of the brain that affect speech or movement, to avoid causing damage. Once the depth electrodes are in place, EEG information is collected directly, a process called electrocorticography. If a single focus is found, the next step may be surgery to remove it. Otherwise only the electrodes themselves are removed.

- **Subdural grid EEG.** This type of EEG involves placing a grid or strip of electrodes on the surface of the brain itself. The electrodes do not enter the brain. The grid system is most frequently used when seizures are in areas affecting language or movement. If a single focus is found, the next step may be surgery to remove it. The grid is usually kept in place for two or more weeks before being removed in a second operation. As with the depth EEG, the scalp will be sore afterwards and will need time to heal thoroughly.

Brain scans

Twenty years ago, neurologists investigating seizure disorders relied on the EEG, patient observation, and possibly risky exploratory surgery to evaluate patients. Today there are other options, including sophisticated brain imaging technologies.

Brain imaging lets doctors take a look inside the skull without doing surgery. They can view tumors and other growths, and they can see whether all of the brain's parts are properly formed. Signs of injury, bleeding, atrophy (brain shrinkage), or disease can be picked up with these tests. It's important to know that even if something abnormal is found, it may not be the cause of the seizures. Minor brain differences are quite common.

Neurologists tend to reserve these tests for cases where a brain injury or tumor is suspected, and for those cases that remain a mystery after one or more EEGs are done. Imaging is used most often when seizures start in adulthood, or when an EEG shows a phenomenon called focal slowing (slower than normal brain activity in a specific location) that could indicate a tumor. If doctors are considering surgery, brain imaging is a must. These techniques may also be used to check brain function after surgery or drug treatment.

The imaging technologies in current use include the following:

- **CT or CAT scan.** Computerized tomography (CT), also called comput-erized axial tomography (CAT), is a computer-enhanced procedure for obtaining x-ray images of the body. Instead of having a fixed x-ray directed at one part of the body, during a CT scan an x-ray tube rotates around the body generating hundreds of images as it moves. These x-ray "slices" are digitized and fed into a computer, which uses them to create two- and three-dimensional pictures. Usually, a special dye is injected into a vein in the arm prior to the procedure. This dye flows to the brain through the circulatory system. CT scans are useful for looking at brain anatomy and can show such things as tumors, tubers (small tumor-like areas of calcification seen in a condition called tuberous sclerosis), areas of damage or atrophy, and structural problems in the brain or its blood vessels. CT scans can only find a definitive seizure focus in about 17 percent of cases. Usually doctors prefer the MRI, unless the patient has a heart pacemaker or another medical device or condition that prevents them from having an MRI.[2]

  Some people are allergic to the dye that's often used during CT scans. If you have a history of allergy or asthma, your neurologist may choose to use a different type of dye or another imaging technology. Aside from the dye injection, the CT scan is painless and risk-free.

- **MRI scan.** Magnetic resonance imaging (MRI) machines use magnets instead of x-rays to create pictures of the brain. These pictures are more detailed than those obtained from a CAT scan, since they detect a sei-zure focus accurately about one-third of the time and produce a more sensitive picture of brain structures.

  When MRI equipment is used properly, accuracy rates of up to 90 per-cent have been reported in cases of temporal lobe epilepsy.[3] You must lie very still inside the MRI machine, which is usually a closed tube, for an accurate picture to be taken. Sometimes an open MRI is available. All

MRI machines make very loud noises, and many people are more comfortable using earplugs.

Steve, age 36, has had two MRIs:

> The main thing is to relax. You can have a blanket if you want, and being warm inside the machine helps. You have to be very still, so get in the most comfortable position you can. The one thing that's distracting is the loud knocking caused by the magnets spinning around. Other than that, it's not too bad.

- **PET scan.** Positron emission tomography (PET) scans measure the distribution of a radioactive tracer in the brain. These radioisotopes, which are given in an injection, are followed with monitoring equipment to reveal patterns of glucose metabolism, as demonstrated by tracing the uptake of a radioactive sugar solution within brain regions. Glucose metabolism (and blood flow, which can be tracked somewhat by following glucose metabolism) is markedly lower than normal in focal areas during the period between seizures, and it rises during a seizure. Other than a minor risk and pain from injection of the radioisotopes, PET scans are not harmful. There is no radiation danger from the radioisotopes. Most PET scanners are located at research hospitals.

- **SPECT scan.** Single photon emission tomography (SPECT) scans can also measure blood flow within the brain. As with PET scans, a tracer material is injected and tracked as it moves through the brain. SPECT scanning done during a seizure is more accurate than scanning between seizures (inter-ictal scanning).[4] A SPECT scan of the brain is sometimes called a neuroSPECT.

Preparing for one of these brain imaging procedures doesn't require you to do anything special: just wear comfortable clothing, leave jewelry and metal hair accessories at home, and be ready to relax. Parents taking children in for imaging may want to bring favorite books, stuffed toys, and the like to keep the child calm and comfortable before the procedure. Parents and spouses can usually stay in the room with the patient if they wish.

Other tests

Your doctor may order a blood test to check your electrolyte levels. Electrolytes are compounds found in blood plasma, within cells, and in body tissues. Essential for proper functioning, they include calcium, potassium, sodium, magnesium, phosphate, and chloride. An imbalance in electrolyte levels can cause seizures and is a clue to underlying health problems. Kidney disease, diabetes, and anorexia are just three of the many medical conditions known to cause electrolyte imbalances.

Other blood tests may also prove helpful, including tests of liver function and checks for vitamin deficiency, lead or other toxic substances, and chemical abnormalities. If hypoglycemia is suspected, your blood glucose level may be checked after an overnight fast. If diabetes is suspected as a cause or complication, your urine will be tested for sugar.

If brain infection is suspected, a spinal tap (also known as a lumbar or spinal puncture) may be ordered to look for signs of infection in the cerebrospinal fluid. A needle is used to extract a small amount of fluid from a space between the third and fourth lumbar vertebrae, located in the lower back. There usually isn't a great deal of pain during the procedure, surprisingly enough, but you may feel sore and tired afterward. Children are more likely to report pain from this procedure, so parents should ask about anesthesia or sedation. There is some risk of infection and fluid leakage. Headache, nausea, and vomiting may also occur after the procedure. Talk to your doctor about things you can do to lower the risk of side effects and about medications that are safe to use in case of nausea.

Your doctor may order a prolactin test, which should be done right after a suspected seizure event. Prolactin is a hormone that is elevated in the blood after most types of epileptic seizures. If prolactin levels right after an event are normal, the person may have something other than epilepsy.

An intracarotid sodium amobarbital test, also known as a Wada test, is sometimes used to help locate speech and memory centers within the brain. The drug sodium amobarbital is injected directly into the carotid artery (in the neck) in such a way that half of the brain is temporarily put to sleep. This lets the doctor run tests of speech, memory, and other functions while the patient can access only one side of her brain. Sometimes an EEG is also done during this procedure. The Wada test is especially crucial before surgery, to ensure that essential areas of the brain are given a wide berth.

Genetic testing is sometimes part of epilepsy diagnosis, especially if an inherited seizure disorder or a developmental disorder characterized by seizures, such as Angelman syndrome or Rett syndrome, is suspected. Identifying and developing tests for genes related to epilepsy is currently the subject of much research. In fact, genetic differences on chromosome 10 have recently been pinpointed as a possible precursor for a type of partial seizure disorder that features auditory auras, and several other areas of the human genome have been linked to an increased risk of certain seizure disorders.[5] Genetic testing is only done if the epilepsy is associated with other signs and symptoms that suggest a syndrome with a known genetic basis.

Genetic testing is usually done on a blood sample. There are two types of tests available. One evaluates the number and structure of the 46 chromosomes for any abnormalities. The second method extracts DNA from cells to look at specific genes. Since each person has 130,000 genes, your medical geneticist or genetic counselor will assist in identifying the correct gene to study. More information on genetic testing is available at http://www.genetests.org.

If a genetic abnormality is found, a genetic counselor will help you learn more about the condition and its prognosis. For information on how to locate a genetic counselor, see Appendix A.

Psychological tests

Psychologists and psychiatrists often use standardized questionnaires and skill tests to screen new patients. These include behavior checklists, developmental scales, and a variety of other instruments. Some tests are screening instruments: simple lists of questions for the patient or the patient's parent that can identify red flags for mental or neurological disorders in general. Others are targeted more precisely, using a battery of questions designed to get information about symptoms of depression.

IQ, speech, and memory tests are also especially helpful for assessing patients who may be having partial seizures. The information gained from tests, if properly administered, can be truly invaluable for ruling out other conditions, making a definitive diagnosis, and designing treatment programs.

Tools for gauging emotional disturbance that ask patients to draw pictures or interpret the pictures or words of others are highly subjective. Some psychologists routinely administer these tests. They include the well-known Rorschach Blot interpretation test, the House-Tree-Person test, and many variations on the same theme.

With children, tests are often administered to rank the individual's development against the norm, usually resulting in a mental age or developmental age score.

Non-epileptic seizures

If you do not have convulsive movements during an episode, and if EEG tests and brain imaging are inconclusive, your neurologist may bring up the possibility of non-epileptic seizures (NES), also known as pseudoseizures. Doctors suspect that people with NES have seizure-like events triggered by something other than abnormal electrical discharge in the brain. The cause may be neurotransmitter imbalances or another chemical problem, creating very real symptoms that closely resemble those of seizures. If you are diagnosed with NES, you needn't feel that you have been labeled a fraud. You simply have a different medical condition. Many people with NES find relief by using medications that affect neurotransmitter production, such as the SSRI (selective serotonin reuptake inhibitor) antidepressants, coupled with therapy to help them cope with their symptoms.

Up to 40 percent of people with epilepsy also have some non-epileptic seizures, usually in the post-ictal period.[6] In such cases, a knowledgeable doctor can work with you to devise strategies for telling the two apart, and for handling both types of events.

Another cause of pseudoseizures is somatization, sometimes called conversion disorder. If you've ever had a worry that caused your stomach to tie itself in knots or made your head pound, you've experienced a common, mild version of this phenomenon—the translation of emotional distress into physical symptoms. Somatization can result in non-epileptic seizures. Some people, particularly women and children, are more prone to somatization. It's important to emphasize that in such cases the seizure-like events are not faked; a poorly understood but very real process in the brain causes them. Treatment is possible and often includes both medication and therapy.

If a doctor discovers that a patient is pretending to have seizures to get attention or special treatment, the diagnosis will be factitious disorder, also known as malingering. (It's important to note that kids with epilepsy, and even some adults, may occasionally fake a seizure for sympathy or to get out of some unwanted chore.) These patients are usually referred to a therapist or psychologist, who can help them learn better techniques for coping with stress, fear, and other emotions.

Many people who have been told that they have pseudoseizures are later more accurately diagnosed as having real seizures. For others, determining the nature of their episodes is simply beyond the current ability of medical science, a frustrating situation for all concerned.

Twelve-year old Richard has Tourette's syndrome and bipolar disorder, and had seizure-like events that for years were labeled as pseudoseizures. Richard was recently diagnosed with a partial seizure disorder after several weeks of intensive testing at a specialist facility. His mother tells about some of their earlier struggles with the diagnostic process:

> He had two big seizures during EEG testing, but they did not show up on the EEG. The epileptologists thought they were pseudoseizures, but the psychiatrists thought they sounded more like real seizures than pseudoseizures. The neurologist at one point commented that there is a very fine line between neurology and psychiatry—and partial seizures, such as Richard may have experienced, fit right along that line. So were these particular episodes true epileptic seizures? Or were they somehow chemically induced via the medications he was taking then? Nobody can give a clear answer to that.

> At this point the neurologist believes most likely something is going awry very deep in Richard's brain, and it will be a matter of luck if we catch it on an EEG. He said that, if this were his son, he would have him on antiseizure meds, because the likelihood that they are real is certainly there.

> We and the school have dramatically reduced any possible stressors for Richard, and we are very careful about medications. His therapist has pointed out that she does not think this is a parenting problem, or a problem in the home, or a traumatic stress problem. She does think they can't give me a single answer because a single answer probably doesn't exist—it could be a combination of his neurological and psychiatric problems, plus a drug interaction.

Diagnosis by elimination

As your neurologist or diagnostic team goes to work, a variety of possibilities may emerge, based on the information gathered. It's important to understand that every medical professional has his own frame of reference. A pediatrician tends to think of parenting and developmental issues. A general practitioner looks at common medical issues first. A psychiatrist thumbs through a book called the *Diagnostic and Statistical Manual of Mental Disorders*, better known as the DSM-IV, for a diagnosis that fits. A neurologist thinks about seizures and brain damage.

It's not feasible for doctors to consider every single possibility, but when the situation is not clear-cut, they need to rule out (or rule in) certain common causes for symptoms. First-year medical students are always taught the old saw, "If you hear hoofbeats, think horses, not zebras." That means that one should consider common problems first when trouble emerges, rather than investigating rare and unusual diseases. It's good basic advice, but some folks really do have stripes! If you or your child do not respond to the usual treatment options, it can be worthwhile to consider other causes, especially if particular symptoms or family history indicate that you should. Doctors call this process *differential diagnosis,* which means finding the right medical label by eliminating others that don't fit.

Looking for seizure causes

Most cases of epilepsy are due to unknown causes. However, depending on the patient's age and the type of seizures he is experiencing, doctors may look for evidence of brain tumor, brain infection, abnormalities of the blood vessels in the brain, problems caused by prescription medication, substance abuse, or other known causes for seizures. If one of these conditions is found, a different treatment route may be needed to control your seizures.

Brain tumors or brain injury

Brain tumors are an important cause of seizures. This cause for seizures is more likely to be considered when epilepsy starts in adulthood.

Brain injury is one of the most common causes for epilepsy that develops after childhood. Penetrating head injury, as from a gunshot wound to the head, is especially likely to result in epilepsy. Closed head wounds, as from a blow to the head or birth trauma, can also result in seizures.[7]

Imaging technologies can help neurologists identify tumors or internal injuries without doing exploratory surgery. Many types of brain tumors can be removed, but a few cannot because of their location or shape. Some tumors that cannot be surgically removed can be treated using radiation and/or medications instead.

Gia tells about her son's experience with seizures secondary to a brain tumor:

> *In the beginning, we didn't know James was having seizures. His were very subtle as a baby, but became more intense and pronounced after surgery. We don't know how much is/was the result of surgery and how much is related to having a moderately sized tumor sitting along his optic tract. We're learning, slowly, to live with them, and work around them.*

Most types of brain injury are allowed to heal on their own. Seizures are sometimes caused by pooling of blood inside the skull or increased pressure on the brain, both of which can be relieved. If the brain injury causes permanent tissue damage or scarring, however, the person may have a seizure disorder even after the initial injury has healed and other symptoms have receded.

Degenerative brain disease and aging

Brain disease is rare in young and middle-aged people, but it is a greater concern for the elderly. Alzheimer's disease, for example, is accompanied by seizure activity about 10 percent of the time. In brain diseases like Alzheimer's, lesions or other abnormal tissue may form and become a seizure focus.[8]

Simply making it past the age of 60 carries some increased risk of seizures, and as the population ages, it's likely that more elderly people will be affected. Partial and complex partial seizures are the most common type of seizures reported in this age group.[9]

It's interesting that seizure medications are playing an increasing role in the treatment of Alzheimer's disease, having shown effectiveness for reducing agitation and aggression in patients with the condition.[10]

Seizures in older patients tend to be the result of stroke or disease, but some may also be medication-induced. Unfortunately, the symptoms of partial or complex partial seizures may be missed in patients who have other serious health problems, or who have difficulty communicating due to degenerative brain disease. Doctors and family members caring for older persons should make themselves knowledgeable about seizure disorders.

Older people who have seizure disorders must exercise extra vigilance about medication interactions. Many of the most widely used medications for conditions affecting the elderly can lower the seizure threshold, and seizure medications can counteract or boost the effects of other medications as well.

Hypoglycemia

Hypoglycemia (low blood sugar) is a deficiency of glucose in the bloodstream. It can cause episodes of confusion, weakness, fainting, sudden loss of energy, and chronic fatigue, all of which could be mistaken for symptoms of partial seizures. If untreated, lack of glucose in the brain can result in seizures, coma, and even death.

To diagnose hypoglycemia, your blood and urine glucose levels will be tested after an overnight fast, and again after drinking a dose of glucose.

Nocturnal hypoglycemia is especially common in people who have insulin-dependent diabetes, particularly those whose treatment regimen is not working as well as it should. Parents of children with diabetes need to be especially vigilant, as children often do not know how to report the feelings associated with hypoglycemia. Indeed, many people with episodes of nocturnal hypoglycemia do not wake up as a result of the episode, leaving them at increased risk of death.

Signs of nocturnal hypoglycemia include insomnia, waking up in a sweat, or waking as a result of strange nightmares, although these symptoms can have many other causes. Diabetes specialists recommend a high-carbohydrate snack at bedtime, coupled with glucose monitoring in the morning. People with nocturnal hypoglycemia may also keep an emergency supply of glucose-rich foods at their bedside to help if they wake suddenly.

Hypoglycemia is also a risk for persons on the ketogenic diet, which is an epilepsy treatment. The ketogenic diet is explained further in Chapter 6, *Other Interventions*.

Infection of the brain

The brain is normally protected from infection, but bacteria and viruses sometimes slip through—especially if the patient has a compromised immune system. The Epstein-Barr virus, human herpes viruses, and many other viruses can cause mood swings, sleep disturbance, psychosis, unusual behavior, and sometimes seizures if they reach the brain.

When brain infection leads to inflammation of brain tissue, it is called encephalitis. Infection of any of the membranes that protect the brain or the spinal cord is known as meningitis. Either of these conditions can lead to seizures.

Blood tests and a spinal tap are the primary tools used to diagnose brain infections. Treatment of nervous system infections depends on which virus or bacteria is the culprit.

If you have particular risk factors for brain infection, such as testing positive for the HIV virus, do not hesitate to talk about them during the epilepsy diagnostic process.

Drug or supplement side effects

Both prescription and over-the-counter medications can cause side effects in some people. Many prescription medicines can lower the seizure threshold, increasing the likelihood of seizures. The list of popular medications that sometimes cause or worsen seizures includes digoxin, Prozac, codeine and other narcotic painkillers, and many more.

Be sure to mention all medications you take, including herbal medicines and vitamin supplements, to your doctor. Even long-term medication users can suddenly experience new side effects. Maturing bodies may react differently to medicines that were previously helpful, tolerance to a medication can change its effects, or a medication's effects may be made stronger by the addition of a second drug.

Over-the-counter (OTC) drugs occasionally implicated in causing or worsening seizures include the following:

- Stimulants like Vivarin and NoDoz
- Stimulant-based diet pills
- Antihistamines containing ephedra, ephedrine, pseudoephedrine, and similar stimulants

The discovery that medication side effects may play a role in the problems a person is experiencing does not rule out a seizure disorder. In fact, some undiagnosed patients "self-medicate" with OTC stimulants, herbal remedies, and other legal substances. Unfortunately, these substances can make the overall situation worse despite seeming to provide temporary relief.

Substance abuse

The use of illegal drugs can produce personality changes, unusual behavior, mood swings, and even psychotic symptoms. Many drugs can cause seizures or make an existing seizure disorder worse. Cocaine and amphetamines are probably the worst offenders.

Alcohol abuse is also a common cause of seizures, especially in alcoholics experiencing withdrawal. Binge drinkers (persons who are not addicted to alcohol but who occasionally or habitually consume large quantities of alcohol in a short period of time) have also been known to have seizures as a result.

Illegal steroids are used far too often, especially by people interested in athletics or bodybuilding. Steroids can cause major mood swings, including both depression and the sudden angry, aggressive behavior that's colloquially known as "roid rage." These episodes could be confused with partial seizures.

Some athletes avoid anabolic steroids and instead use other substances that supposedly enhance performance but also lower the seizure threshold, such as stimulants or even insulin.

Substance abuse can also be a symptom of epilepsy, however, as people who are disturbed by their symptoms may find that drinking or doing drugs masks their discomfort for a little while. For that reason, the discovery that a patient has been abusing drugs or alcohol does not rule out a diagnosis of a seizure disorder.

Ken, who now works as an advocate for people with epilepsy, tells how his scary symptoms turned him toward substance abuse as a teenager:

> In May of 1985, I was an honor roll student, on the debate team, and beginning to weight lift. I was going to have to lose 40 pounds to meet the criteria for competition, so I went to school at 7:45 every morning and worked out for an hour and started a "banana and milk" diet. One day I was leaving class to go to lunch, and a strange feeling came over me. For some reason I couldn't understand, I turned the wrong way as I left the room. The next thing I knew, I was in the parking lot of the high school, at the very opposite end of the school from where I should have been. I remember feeling very confused, and thinking the diet must have caused me to have a blackout. I didn't dare tell anyone, because I thought I might have to quit the diet. Over the summer, the blackouts kept happening;

strange, short bursts of altered perception started; and within four or five months, they increased to as many as four a day.

I started becoming very introverted, thinking I was somehow "crazy." My marks dropped, I became very argumentative, and I had no social life. I watched TV a lot and began to create delusions about my directing videos I watched and being part of shows. My friends remember me obsessing about expensive cars and other material things. As my GPA dropped, my parents began disciplining me. I found it much easier to drift off into the fantasy world. I also began sneaking alcohol into my bedroom.

One night my parents asked me to sit down at the kitchen table with them. They asked me what was making my grades drop, my temper get bad, and avoid driving. I told them about the blackouts, and I was taken to the doctor. I expected it to be some diet problem. He suggested it might be epilepsy, and I went to a neurologist, where I was diagnosed nearly two years after my seizures began. I now wonder how no one noticed the seizures. My automatisms are so obvious, someone must have noticed.

The delusions took almost three years to overcome—I had a problem with alcohol and drugs again in 1988 due to the frustration. Late in 1989 I was referred to a new epileptologist who has been a great help ever since. It has been a very long 15 years, and I still have about ten partial complex seizures and one partial simple a month, but it's been a challenge that has taught me much.

Although it can be embarrassing to reveal that you use illegal drugs or have a problem with alcohol, it is absolutely essential to tell your neurologist. These behaviors may or may not be causing your seizures, but they can definitely affect your treatment and your general quality of health.

Help is readily available for both addiction and abuse, and it's preferable to access that help as early as possible, before the problem gets too big to handle or has legal or medical consequences. Even if drug or alcohol abuse has continued for many years, there are effective treatment options available.

Vascular abnormalities

Abnormalities or disease in the brain's veins and arteries (vascular problems) can also cause seizures, although this is a rare phenomenon in younger patients. The older a person is when epilepsy begins, the more likely that vascular problems or stroke are the cause. Stroke is the most common cause of new-onset seizures in the elderly.

The two vascular abnormalities most likely to cause seizures in younger adults are arteriovenous malformations (AVMs) or cavernous malformations (cavernous angiomas, or cavernomas). AVMs are unusually shaped veins or arteries. They change how blood flows within the brain, raising blood pressure and causing an increased risk of hemorrhaging, tissue damage, lesion formation, and seizures. A cavernoma is a lesion (an area of injury or damage) within brain tissue. The lesion itself can cause seizure activity, and its presence increases the chance of hemorrhage within the brain, which could also cause seizures. MRI imaging is used to diagnose these problems.[11]

If one of these types of vascular abnormalities is found, surgery is usually performed as soon as possible. Treatment for stroke includes reducing risks for additional strokes by changing diet and other lifestyle factors, rehabilitation to address the affects of the stroke, and medication if indicated (for example, if the stroke was related to high blood pressure, as many are).

Comorbid conditions and seizure mimics

Some people have both a partial seizure disorder and another health problem, perhaps one of several conditions that occur slightly more frequently in people who have epilepsy. Diagnoses that exist alongside your primary condition of epilepsy are called comorbid conditions. They may or may not affect the symptoms of or treatment for seizures.

Although your neurologist will focus his attention on seizures, it's also important to consider all facets of a patient's health and development. This ensures that the final diagnosis is accurate and that treatments for disparate conditions do not conflict with each other.

There are also a few medical conditions whose symptoms could mimic a partial seizure disorder. The following sections describe some of the medical and neuropsychiatric conditions your doctor may look at while she attempts to pinpoint a diagnosis.

Anxiety disorders

Anxiety disorders are common enough that almost everyone knows someone who suffers from one. They include panic disorders and extreme phobias of all sorts, from claustrophobia (fear of being in small, enclosed places) to arachnophobia (fear of spiders). Simply put, they all involve an extreme reaction to certain situations or stimuli, as the body puts its "fight or flight" system in motion for no good reason.

Some people with anxiety disorders have panic attacks so severe that they could almost be mistaken for seizures. They may make rapid movements, have an increased heartbeat, hyperventilate, or even pass out. EEG and brain imaging evidence should help your doctor make a definitive diagnosis.

On the other hand, some people experience sudden feelings of dread, panic, or fear during a seizure. Partial seizures—especially undiagnosed ones—can also be a source of anxiety and fear after the fact.

Some people suffer from both seizures and anxiety, and repeated seizures can even lead to a form of post-traumatic stress disorder (PTSD), which can be described as a cumulative neurophysical reaction to one or more frightening events. Medication and counseling can help people overcome anxiety disorders, including PTSD.

Attention Deficit Disorder

The hyperactivity that most of us think of as part and parcel of Attention Deficit Hyperactivity Disorder (ADHD) is not a symptom of partial seizure disorders. However, if the first symptom reported is having trouble paying attention or daydreaming, the "inattentive type" of ADHD—usually called Attention Deficit Disorder (ADD)—may be considered.

The DSM-IV criteria for ADD requires six or more of the following symptoms, persisting for at least six months, occurring frequently, and occurring to a degree inconsistent with the child's developmental level:

- Fails to pay attention to details; makes careless mistakes in schoolwork or other activities
- Has difficulty sustaining attention in schoolwork, chores, or play activities
- Does not seem to listen when spoken to directly
- Fails to follow instructions; does not finish schoolwork or chores (but not due to deliberate oppositional behavior or failure to understand instructions)
- Has difficulty organizing tasks and activities

- Avoids, dislikes, or is reluctant to try tasks that require sustained mental effort, such as homework
- Loses things needed for tasks or activities, such as toys, homework assignments, or books
- Is easily distracted by noise or other external stimuli
- Is forgetful in daily activities

When you read these criteria, it's easy to see how someone with a partial seizure disorder could be misdiagnosed with ADD. The main difference is that seizures change behavior in episodes, not all the time. However, if a person is having many partial or complex seizures during the day, it can be hard to see the episodic pattern. Careful observation, EEG testing, and brain imaging may be used to rule in or rule out partial or absence seizures.

Bipolar disorders

Bipolar disorders are characterized by mood swings that may include depression, hypomania (extreme elation), mania (very extreme elation and agitation), and normalcy. Both epilepsy and bipolar disorders can include auras, and both appear to include a kindling-like process in which episodes start with some sort of internal stimulus or event that begins a cascade of processes. Although thought disorders are more common in bipolar disorders, they are also sometimes seen in people with temporal lobe epilepsy or other types of partial seizures.

The main difference between these two conditions is the length of episodes. Partial seizures are usually brief, lasting from a few seconds to a few minutes, while mood swings can last for months. The exceptions to this rule are bipolar patients who are "rapid cyclers." These patients may experience dozens of wild mood swings in a single day. They are also more likely than non-rapid-cyclers to have EEG abnormalities.

It can be harder to tell some types of partial seizures from bipolar episodes than one might expect, unless conclusive evidence is found to rule in or rule out seizures via an EEG or brain imaging. Sometimes doctors must work with their best guess and simply try treatments until one seems to help. The best-known medication for bipolar disorders is lithium, a naturally occurring mineral salt. If lithium does not work, several drugs normally used for epilepsy are also considered first-line treatments for bipolar patients.

Central auditory processing disorder

Central auditory processing disorder (CAPD) affects how the brain processes sound and speech. A person with CAPD may appear to be oblivious to sound or unable to pay attention. For young children with CAPD, speech may not make sense, and speech delays and disorders occur.

As with ADD, the main difference between CAPD and seizures is that seizures are episodic, not constant. EEG testing and brain imaging can be used to rule in or rule out partial or absence seizures.

Developmental disorders

Seizure disorders are much more common in persons who have autistic spectrum disorders, mental retardation, and other developmental disorders than they are in the general population. These conditions may be caused by the same genetic factors that cause some types of seizures, or by brain damage or infection that also causes seizures (indeed, before the advent of reliable medications for seizure control, untreated epilepsy was a leading cause of mental retardation). Epilepsy and developmental disorders are, however, separate conditions—and under no circumstances should anyone accept lack of seizure treatment simply because a person also has a developmental delay or disorder. The presence of uncontrolled seizures can only slow development even more, impair quality of life, and increase the person's risk for early death. Treatment of comorbid seizure disorders, on the other hand, often leads to developmental progress and an improved quality of life for persons with developmental disorders.

Diabetes

Diabetes is a family of metabolic disorders that have autoimmune and genetic components. People with diabetes are unable to use carbohydrates and sugars efficiently to produce energy, due to insufficiency or lack of insulin, a pancreatic hormone. The result is high blood sugar (hyperglycemia). The body tries to use fats as an energy source instead, but the by-products of metabolizing fats (ketones) build up in the bloodstream. Symptoms of uncontrolled diabetes can include mood swings, lightheadedness, frequent urination, fainting, seizures, and even diabetic coma and death (see the section "Hypoglycemia" earlier in this chapter).

In the US, about 6 percent of the population suffers from some form of diabetes. The rate is highest among persons of African, Asian, Hispanic, or Native American ancestry. The risk of developing diabetes increases with age, obesity, and physical inactivity.

Diabetes should be considered as a potential cause of seizure-like episodes if a person has other risk factors. Also, anyone with diabetes and a tendency toward seizures should ensure that they have a good treatment team to work with, including at minimum a doctor (preferably a diabetes management specialist or endocrinologist) and a dietitian.

Hormonal disorders

Hormones are chemicals secreted in one part of the body that control or influence activity in another part of the body. Although there are quite a few types of hormones, the best-known hormones are testosterone and estrogen, which our bodies produce in varied amounts according to our gender and age.

Most hormones are secreted by one of the several glands that make up the endocrine system, including the thyroid, adrenal, and pituitary glands; the pancreas; and the testes and ovaries.

If there's a problem with the endocrine system, that problem may also affect the production, transmission, or use of neurotransmitters like serotonin and dopamine. This may be one of the reasons that seizures tend to emerge, worsen, or improve (depending on the patient) just before or during periods of special hormonal activity, such as menstruation, puberty, the transition from adolescence to adulthood, pregnancy, the period just after giving birth, and menopause. In some patients, hormonal problems may mimic the symptoms of seizure disorders. In others, they may be intimately intertwined. Getting treatment for an underlying hormonal disorder has contributed greatly to the stability of many people with seizures. Of course, some medications used to treat hormonal disorders can also lower the seizure threshold.

Some women experience seizures in concert with their menstrual cycle, a variant known as catamenial epilepsy.

Hormonal disorders that mimic or contribute to seizure activity can usually be identified with blood tests and can often be treated with hormone supplements. Some women will find relief by taking birth control pills, having injections of Depo-Provera, or getting Norplant implants.

Steroid medications, such as prednisone, also have a place in epilepsy treatment because of the influence of hormonal activity on seizures. They are most commonly used in cases of childhood epilepsy that do not respond to other medications. See Chapter 5, *Medical Interventions*, for more information about hormones and steroids as a treatment option.

Intermittent explosive disorder

Intermittent explosive disorder (IED) is a diagnostic label for people who have sudden outbursts of anger or rage. Since this can also be a symptom of a partial seizure disorder, if that behavior is observed during or (more commonly) just after a seizure, the IED label might be used until other evidence of epilepsy is found. Some studies of people diagnosed with IED suggest that seizures or seizure-like activity may underlie most cases of this disorder, while other experts argue that the underlying problem is an impulse-control disorder.

Episodic dyscontrol syndrome, sometimes colloquially known as limbic rage, is a label used to describe aggressive episodes believed to derive from dysregulation of the brain's limbic system. This regulatory problem may or may not have a relationship to seizure activity.

Neurologists say that sudden rages are actually one of the most common reasons for adults to wonder if they might have a partial seizure disorder. However, it's fairly rare for this to be the case. Sudden rages are far more likely to indicate the presence of a bipolar disorder and are sometimes also seen in people with Tourette's syndrome or related disorders.

Migraine

Migraine is a common, chronic, and painful condition experienced by about one in five women and one in twenty men. Migraine headaches—blinding, temple-pounding events that may be preceded by an aura and that may last for hours—are only the best-known manifestation of migraine. Many migraine sufferers also experience stomach pains, nausea, sudden sensitivity to light and sound, and other intensely uncomfortable sensations.

Jane, age 35, had a history of migraines that caused her to delay seeking a diagnosis:

About six years ago, I started having migraines preceded by trembling/shaking of the right arm that lasted from a few seconds to several minutes. I treated these as migraine auras. (I had what doctors called migraines for a long time prior to this.) About four years ago, my right leg started "bouncing" intermittently for a few seconds to several minutes. This usually happened on the way to or from work, and it would usually go away if I concentrated on driving or used the leg. Occasionally when walking, the leg would buckle under me.

In the past 18 months or so, just before falling asleep, I'd hear what I call a "zing," starting in one ear and going through my brain to the other ear. Imagine the sound your computer monitor makes when you first turn it on—that's a zing. After hearing the zing, I'd be wide awake. Then I started having what I call "brain shifts." To me, these feel like two parts of the brain are sliding against each other for a split second. The feeling originates just left of the center of my brain. Some of them are so bad, my head actually jerks. A few months before going to the doctor, I started having occasions where I'd stumble around like I was drunk, and my speech would slur. I also started having problems finding words when I spoke, and problems typing (really annoying when typing is a huge part of your job).

I either ignored all these problems, or attributed them to being tired or growing older. Never went to the doctor for any of them, and sure didn't associate them with each other.

On the day I was diagnosed, I was having a particularly bad episode of trembles in my right arm that just wouldn't stop, then my right leg started, and then my whole right side got involved. One of my co-workers finally convinced me to go to the doctor, immediately.

My GP thought it was probably related to migraines, but called a neuro, just in case—thank you, Doc! The neuro ordered an EEG, which came back positive for seizure activity. The MRI they ordered next was negative for any tumors, scars, etc. A second EEG and a 24-hour EEG were both positive, and so I was diagnosed with complex partial seizures, originating in the left temporal lobe. I was almost happy to get a diagnosis—all my problems were finally starting to worry me, and epilepsy could explain most of them.

Migraine is caused by differences within the central nervous system that can be inherited and that, like seizures, are impacted by hormonal activity. The exact mechanism of migraine is still not fully understood, but it is believed to include changes in the amount or use of the neurotransmitters serotonin and noradrenaline, which then affect blood flow in the brain.

A person having a migraine attack does not lose consciousness, but can have some seizure-like symptoms, including auras and difficulty with moving, seeing, or speaking. Another difference between migraine and seizure is obvious: pain. In addition, migraine does not cause seizure patterns on an EEG, although the muscle-tensing that often accompanies a migraine can produce artifacts on the readout.

Migraine is more common in people with any type of seizure disorder, and vice versa. It is highest among those people with epilepsy that's secondary to a head trauma. Interestingly, almost half of people with epilepsy who have migraine symptoms are never diagnosed, possibly because epilepsy diagnosis and treatment have taken precedence over looking at other health concerns, but also because the symptoms can be similar.[12]

Migraine treatment requires a combination of lifestyle changes (such as avoiding migraine-triggering foods and reducing stress) and medication. When all other medications have failed to prevent debilitating migraine attacks, anti-epilepsy drugs are often tried. It is likely that these medications help by preventing the migraine kindling process, even though it is not identical to the seizure kindling process.

Personality disorders

There are two major ways of looking at personality disorders. The official view is that they are ways of seeing the world, reacting to events, and relating to people that are maladaptive and that cause problems for the people who have them. Most psychiatrists believe that personality disorders arise from childhood difficulties and conflicts, so they are rarely diagnosed in young children. Symptoms must be present by early adulthood, however. A second view is that personality disorders are, at least in part, mild versions or "shadows" of major biologically based mental or neurological disorders.

The DSM-IV identifies eleven major personality disorders (PDs), which it divides into three groups: Clusters A, B, and C (or I, II, and III). Some doctors believe that personality disorders are more common in people with epilepsy. It's unknown whether that's because some children with seizures miss out on healthy personality development due to their illness, or because some personality characteristics are determined by the same genes or other influences that can cause epilepsy. In fact, the whole personality disorder/epilepsy connection is controversial and unproven.

Very briefly defined, the personality disorders are the following:

- Cluster A

    - **Paranoid**. Distrustful; suspicious of others and their motives.

    - **Schizoid**. Very limited social and emotional range.

    - **Schizotypal**. Limited social and emotional range coupled with unusual thought and behavior patterns.

- Cluster B

    - **Antisocial**. Unconcerned about rules, laws, or the rights of others; often violent, aggressive, and destructive. Also called sociopathic or psychopathic personality.

    - **Borderline**. Unstable relationships, values, self-image, and emotions; reckless and impulsive; episodes of aggressive or highly emotional behavior.

    - **Histrionic**. Attention-seeking; highly emotional.

    - **Narcissistic**. Self-absorbed, self-important, and demanding; limited understanding of other people's perspectives.

- Cluster C

    - **Avoidant**. Feels inadequate; overly sensitive to criticism; avoids social interaction.

    - **Dependent**. Overly dependent on others for approval or care; clinging and submissive.

    - **Obsessive-Compulsive**. Overly controlled (and controlling), orderly, and perfectionistic.

You may hear about other personality disorders that are not currently listed in the DSM-IV. One of these is depressive personality disorder, which can be defined as having a chronically gloomy outlook on life without being clinically depressed. Another is passive-aggressive personality disorder, which involves using passive resistance to express anger (for example, playing the long-suffering martyr rather than telling your husband off). To ensure that any other personality problems have a clinical label, some psychiatrists may employ the term "personality disorder, not otherwise specified."

Schizoaffective disorder

The terms schizoaffective disorder or schizoaffective depression indicate that the patient has some characteristics of a mood disorder, such as a bipolar disorder, and some characteristics of schizophrenia. This diagnosis is sometimes accidentally applied to people with undiagnosed partial or complex partial seizures. See the sections "Bipolar disorders" and "Schizophrenia" for characteristics that help doctors tell the difference between those disorders and seizure disorders.

Schizophrenia

Schizophrenia is a major mental illness characterized by psychotic symptoms, often including complete loss of connection with reality. Because a person having a partial or complex partial seizure also experiences alteration of consciousness, it's not at all unusual for the patient or her family to fear that they are seeing early signs of schizophrenia. People sometimes make repetitive movements during partial seizures that could also be confused with the repetitive (stereotypic) movements made by some people with schizophrenia.

One big difference between schizophrenia and epilepsy involves what psychiatrists call "affect": schizophrenics are usually said to have a blunt affect, meaning that they're apathetic about what's going on around them, and they lack much "personality."

Another difference is that seizures are sudden and episodic, while schizophrenia almost always has a slow, gradually worsening onset. It also does not normally wax and wane.

A third difference is that schizophrenics are more likely to suffer from a thought disorder. While patients in either group may have hallucinatory or delusional experiences, the person who has just had a partial seizure is likely to realize that the phenomena he experienced during it were not real. The schizophrenic person is not connected enough with objective reality to tell the difference between reality and fantasy. Schizophrenics are also more likely to have truly bizarre delusions, including psychotic symptoms that don't jibe with their outward mood. For example, they may seem quite cheerful while informing you that the walls are dripping with blood.

EEG and brain imaging evidence may be inconclusive. In cases where differential diagnosis is difficult, it's sometimes accidentally made via medication: schizophrenia does not respond to anti-epilepsy drugs, and epilepsy does not respond to the neuroleptic drugs most useful for schizophrenia.

Of course, a person can have both epilepsy and schizophrenia.

Syncope

Syncope is a fancy medical word for fainting. There are all sorts of reasons for fainting. One of the most common is a sudden drop in blood pressure, as one might experience when standing up too quickly from a lying or sitting position. In susceptible people, syncope can be triggered by anything from defecation to fear. Some people even have automatism-like movements while in a faint, a variant known as convulsive syncope. Careful observation and an EEG should clear up any confusion between a faint and a true seizure.

Tuberous sclerosis

Tuberous sclerosis is a rare condition in which tiny, tumor-like fingers of tissue grow inside the brain, and often in the heart, kidneys, eyes, and on the skin. Some people with tuberous sclerosis have seizures and may also have autistic features and/or mental retardation. Persons with this disorder generally have a genetic abnormality on chromosome 9 or chromosome 16.

Commonly it is seizures that first bring a person with tuberous sclerosis to a neurologist. Brain imaging identifies the tubers, and other signs are found in a neurological workup.

Unipolar depression

Unipolar, or "simple," depression is just that: depressed mood that lasts longer than two weeks and is not due to another medical condition, the side effects of medication, or normal reaction to a major life event (such as grieving after a parent's death). It is the most common form of depression.

Since mood swings can be caused by seizures, particularly in temporal lobe epilepsy, it's not unusual for an adult with partial seizures to first seek help during or because of a depressive episode. Doctors may then prescribe one of the anti-depressant drugs commonly used to treat unipolar depression: selective serotonin reuptake inhibitors (SSRIs) such as Paxil, Prozac, and Effexor; or tricyclic anti-depressants, such as Anafranil or Tofranil. Unfortunately, all of these drugs can lower the seizure threshold for some people, occasionally revealing the presence of undiagnosed epilepsy.

The presence of depression certainly does not rule out a seizure disorder; in fact, depression is much more common in people with epilepsy, including both children and adults.[13]

The waiting game

It may take a while for your neurologist to come to a conclusion. This can be frustrating, but it's much better than having a doctor jump to conclusions! While you wait, seek counseling if you feel it might help you stay calm and cope with your symptoms. It can be very useful to talk to someone who is knowledgeable and nonjudgmental about the difficulties you face.

Don't let yourself be frightened by any of the remote possibilities that may be considered during the diagnostic process. Despite the seriousness of many health conditions that can mimic or cause seizures, most of them are eminently treatable, as are partial seizure disorders.

Of course, if you have any reason to believe that you or your child is in danger—for example, if symptoms have contributed to dangerous falls, created problems while driving or performing hazardous work, or caused you to consider suicide—you shouldn't be forced to wait for months to get relief. It's often possible to treat symptoms without knowing for certain what the final diagnosis will be. Day treatment and hospitalization are also options that can keep you safe if finding a diagnosis takes a long time.

The diagnostic report

Once your neurologist and any additional team members have completed all observations, interviews, and testing, it will be time to make a diagnosis. This is usually done in a report that describes the patient; summarizes the events, observations, and tests that led up to the diagnosis; and finally presents the doctor's diagnosis. Most practitioners will also include suggestions for therapy, medications, or schooling based on what was learned.

For most patients, the diagnosis will be fairly short: simple partial seizures, complex partial seizures, tonic-clonic seizures, or some combination of these three types. Occasionally evidence from EEGs, brain imaging, and observation will indicate a specific type of epilepsy that can be differentiated in some way from others. If you or your child is diagnosed with one of these conditions (several of which are listed in the Glossary), there may be special treatments available. All of the specific epilepsy syndromes are relatively rare; some of them are extraordinarily so.

Some people interviewed for this book noted that they were never given a copy of the final diagnostic report. Instead, they may have been informed of the diagnosis verbally—even over the phone—without getting much information or a chance to ask questions. Seizure disorders are chronic medical conditions that can be hard to treat. A good diagnostician knows that a label alone isn't much help. It must be accompanied by information about what should happen next, and what you can expect in the future. Be sure to ask for copies of any reports, including scores on standardized tests and imaging results. If your diagnosing professional isn't forthcoming with this level of information, move on to someone else who is more committed to working closely with you.

If the diagnostic report is hard to read, an advocate from your nearest epilepsy group, a therapist, or a social worker may be able to help. These people have a background in medical jargon and the mumbo-jumbo of testing, and they can translate it into "real-world" language for you.

One thing that may be missing from the diagnostic report is a prognosis. Doctors are often reluctant to give this information—after all, they can't predict the future, and they don't want to raise false hopes or dash high ones. Still, this is information you need to make good choices about future medical care. Simply explain that you want to know about the usual course and outcome of the type of seizure disorder found, and what might be possible with the treatments recommended or with other types of treatments.

You may want to schedule a follow-up appointment specifically to discuss your condition and your neurologist's treatment recommendations. Write down any questions you have. If time is limited, ask your doctor if you can call or email with any questions that might be left over.

CHAPTER 3

Living with Partial Seizure Disorders

Simply getting a diagnosis and understanding the symptoms of partial seizure disorders makes these conditions easier to cope with, but other people don't always understand. This chapter discusses some of the most common challenges that partial seizure disorders pose for patients and their families, and it talks about ways that others have successfully handled them. Topics include other people's perceptions of epilepsy, dealing with problems at work and in the community, and having children.

Parents and teenagers may also want to consult Chapter 4, *Growing Up with Partial Seizure Disorders*, for information about developmental delays, special education, and other issues of particular importance to children.

The effect that seizures have on your life depends on many variables, including your age at onset, what kind of work you do or want to do, your life goals, your personal value system, and the culture that you live within. Some people with very severe, frequent seizures feel that they have a wonderful quality of life despite their medical challenges, because they have good relationships, social acceptance, and work or other activities that make them feel happy and productive. Some people whose seizures are much less debilitating feel that they have a poor quality of life because of discrimination, lack of acceptance by friends and family members, or a self-pitying attitude.

If your seizure disorder prevents you from reaching personal goals—for example, if you are an airline pilot and lose your ability to work at a job you love because of adult-onset epilepsy—it's natural to feel upset. Combating discrimination and stigma is also time-consuming and depressing. No matter how your seizures affect you physically or mentally, you can't control other people's reactions and opinions. You can only choose to maintain a positive outlook, search for opportunities to reach new goals, and educate or ignore those who are not supportive. You have allies, including other people with epilepsy (remember, that's about 1 in every 100 people) and, in many cases, public opinion and the law.

Dealing with stigma

It's hard to believe that, within living memory, many medical doctors thought seizures were caused by character defects or emotional problems. Outside of the medical community, ideas about epilepsy were even stranger. There are still many cultures in which seizures are believed to be a form of demonic possession or are given another otherworldly explanation. People with epilepsy have historically been denied access to many types of jobs and discriminated against socially as a direct result of these false beliefs.

Rebecca, age 41, says the stigma attached to seizure disorders has affected her strongly:

> I spend a lot of time in fear, as I have been told things like "control yourself," "you gotta overcome that," "you should be questioning your salvation," and "you're so selfish," etc. I have lost friends over epilepsy, so I am gun-shy around people.

> My college told me I needed to "leave for a year and come back when you've got it together, and have a doctor's permission" when I had undiagnosed seizures in the classroom in 1979. I finished in the fall of 1982 via make up work. The college really put out for me—and I am grateful, even though my condition prevented me from getting the professional job (counselor) I had trained for. The education proved valuable in my present job.

Remnants of old attitudes still haunt people with seizure disorders, and people who have partial seizures also have to cope with negative attitudes about mental illness, since some people have never heard of having seizures without convulsions and instead assume that the person is "crazy."

Many uninformed people do not comprehend that the brain is simply another organ of the body, like the stomach, lungs, or heart. Just as heart disease affects that organ's primary function of pumping blood through the body, illness or injury to the brain affects its primary function of thought and cognition. Brain malfunctions have no more connection with your innate moral character or personal worth than heart malfunctions. It's unfair for anyone with an illness affecting the brain to be misjudged or dismissed as insane, whether the root cause of their symptoms is a viral illness, schizophrenia, depression, or a partial seizure disorder, but it's a reality. Until most people understand and accept the concept of biologically based brain disorders, it will be uncomfortable for many patients with partial seizures to talk about some of their symptoms.

In 1997, the World Health Organization (WHO) launched an epilepsy awareness campaign in concert with the International League Against Epilepsy and the International Bureau for Epilepsy. Its goal was to build public perception of seizure disorders as treatable medical problems. The campaign faced an uphill battle, according to WHO: recent studies indicate that three-fourths of people with epilepsy get no treatment for the condition, with that figure rising to 90 percent in the developing world.

When you look at WHO's data, it's easy to understand why a person might not seek a diagnosis and treatment. For example, in China and India, epilepsy is legal grounds for annulling a marriage—in fact, 72 percent of Chinese adults surveyed would object if their child wished to marry someone with epilepsy, and 31 percent felt that such individuals should not hold jobs, either.[1]

The level of stigma attached to seizure disorders depends on where you live, of course. A 1998 survey of patients in fifteen European countries found that slightly over half believed that the disorder made them less acceptable socially, with 18 percent feeling strongly stigmatized. The degree of personal negative perceptions correlated with how difficult one's seizures were to control and cope with, and there were large differences in how people from various countries felt.[2]

Self-perceived stigma, even comments and stares from others, are hard enough to handle. Until recently, however, discrimination against persons with any known handicap was both common and legal. Many would argue that it is still common, and in some countries it remains legal as well.

Throughout history, people with epilepsy have been affected by laws that prevent them from enjoying a variety of everyday activities, from joining the military or attaining a security clearance, to marrying and having children. In the US, laws mandating sterilization and/or institutionalization of people with epilepsy existed in some states as late as the 1950s, and some physicians still suggest sterilization today.

Both Western nations and many countries in Africa, Asia, and Latin America now have laws intended to prevent discrimination against people with disabilities. Unfortunately, even in the US, which is acknowledged as having the strongest set of anti-discrimination statutes in the world, people with brain disorders frequently discover that they are not given the same protection as people with visible physical disabilities.

Disabled people in general experience housing, work, and social discrimination, and those who have mobility, sensory, or communications impairments often find that their needs are simply not taken into account (a form of de facto discrimination that limits their participation in society).

Damaged self-esteem is one result of discrimination, but embarrassment and misplaced shame aren't the main reasons people hide the fact that they have seizures or hide the severity of their seizures. It's the public policy results of stigma, such as revocation of a license to drive, that are most likely to encourage secrecy. A British study found that one-sixth of people with epilepsy hid the disorder from their physician, or understated its severity, to prevent loss of their driving privileges and jobs. Their fears are not without basis: according to the study's author, 17 percent of people who concealed their seizure disorder in the UK are unemployed, but a full 47 percent who do not conceal it are without work.[3]

When you are faced with discrimination based on ignorance, it's important to stand your ground, whether or not you have the backing of civil rights laws like the Americans with Disabilities Act. One of the most important things that anyone with a seizure disorder can do is to inform themselves fully about their condition, making it easier to use facts to answer any questions that come up. Simply having that knowledge base helps you feel comfortable with talking about your seizures and how they affect you, and with defending yourself against people who are rude or just ignorant.

Self-advocacy gives you power in the workplace, at school, and in social relationships. Many people tend to feel uncomfortable with this duty, but it is crucial. Getting involved in groups like the Epilepsy Foundation or parent advocacy organizations often goes a long way toward increasing your level of comfort and courage. It also gives you a chance to advocate for others who may not be as far along that path as you are—newly diagnosed people, children, and elderly patients, for example.

For more information about epilepsy and discrimination, see "Epilepsy and your rights" later in this chapter. The Epilepsy Foundation also provides a very thorough guide on the Web at *http://www.efa.org/advocacy/legal.html* and has a brochure on this topic, *The Legal Rights of Persons with Epilepsy* (see Appendix A, *Resources*).

Seizures in public

Stigma and courage collide when it comes to the problem of having seizures in public. For those who have tonic-clonic seizures, the issues are obvious—you may fall and get hurt, people may gather around and stare, and some well-meaning but misguided individual may think you'll bite your tongue and try to put something in your mouth, hold you down, or call for an ambulance. One thing is certain: people will see your convulsions and know that you are having a seizure.

If your seizures don't include convulsions, however, they may think you're "spaced out," on drugs, drunk, or mentally ill—and you may be in no state to defend yourself against their ignorance and its fallout. That's why so many people with partial seizures have learned to quickly remove themselves from social situations when they feel those familiar presentiments of an episode coming on.

Cheri, age 29, says that being prepared is the best way to cope with the possibility of seizures in public:

> If I am not at work, sitting out my seizures is the safest course. The partials are very internal, and though my family members are able to recognize them quite well through breathing patterns and so on, I had one in front of my neurologist and he couldn't tell anything had happened. I work full-time at a grocery store, however, and there it is a different matter. When a problem is recognized by a customer or another worker, someone must take over the checkstand where I am working and get me out of the way. I've simply asked to be taken somewhere quiet where I can sit down and get my mind in working order, and then we go on from there. I used to wear a bracelet, but tended to change medications more rapidly than I could update the bracelet. I do wear a leather pouch around my neck holding the magnet that can initiate my vagus nerve stimulator. I have informed a great number of people at work and church how to use it, but it is mainly for added peace of mind. The magnet is almost never used. I can see why people whose seizures are uncommon might not share their situation with others, but that's just not sensible for me. It's better for everyone there if the best responses are made known up front.
>
> While I try not to let my epilepsy change what I do every day and the way I act around people, that doesn't mean it doesn't strongly affect my

lifestyle. My home has been chosen within walking distance of stores where I was already working or could transfer to, because my insurance has been essential for both my health and my husband's. If my husband ever needs a ride (car lube, eyes being tested, and so forth), I'm not the one who can provide it, because of the valid concern I and everyone else have about a possible seizure behind the wheel. Soon he will have surgery and others must come to help him around. I don't feel that I am less of a person due to my epilepsy, but I do sometimes feel very helpless and dependent. Nonetheless, I have long believed that your biggest problem in life is your attitude toward your problems, and I try continually to keep my attitude high.

However, it's not always possible, or desirable, to go into hiding when a seizure is imminent. A strong argument can be made for having the right to have symptoms in public, visible or invisible—if they make other people uncomfortable, the problem is really theirs.

The healthiest attitude is probably a pragmatic one. Learn to recognize your triggers, early warning signs, and auras, and plan where to go and what to do in advance, based on your personal preferences and the options available. Think through typical scenarios based on where you might be—at home, at work, at school, in a store, on the bus, or behind the wheel of your car.

If you have the time and opportunity to get yourself to a comfortable, safe place, do so if you wish. You may want to alert a friend, family member, or coworker. Chapter 6, *Other Interventions*, includes a variety of self-help ideas suggested by other people with partial seizure disorders and by medical professionals. These tools may help you avoid or shorten the length of your seizures, reducing your fear of having a public episode. Some people are able to use certain medications to truncate episodes as well.

It's a good idea to inform several trusted people about how to handle your seizures in case one occurs in public, at school, or on the job. That way you have an advocate who can reliably speak for you when necessary. If your workplace or your child's school has a nurse on-site or a person assigned to respond to medical emergencies, make sure this person has all of the necessary information. Items they should know include:

- Your diagnosis
- Medications you take

- How to respond during a seizure (including a tonic-clonic seizure, even if you have never had one before)

- When and where to call for medical help (including your doctor's phone number and the name and address of your hospital of choice)

- Your health insurance information

If, on the other hand, you are among strangers and there's nowhere to go when a seizure hits, it's a good thing to have a medical alert bracelet or, better yet, a card that explains what's going on and how you would like people to respond. Your card's wording will depend on the characteristics of your seizures, of course. A sample card might read:

> *I have complex partial seizures that sometimes temporarily prevent me from speaking and reacting normally. I would appreciate it if you could help me find a place to sit down, and then call my friend Joe at 123-4567. There is no need to call an ambulance.*

If you have a chance to hand the card to someone, such as a security guard or shopkeeper, great. If you don't, make sure one is easy to find in your purse or wallet, just in case an ambulance or the police are called. People who live in communities where languages other than English are commonly spoken may want to have this card translated, just in case.

Pat says she always carries a medical alert card in case of public emergencies:

> *I carry an information card because I've had seizures in public. I believe people who have found me have used the card to call paramedics. I once had a seizure in Central Park in New York City and someone dug through my bag, found the card, and called an ambulance (and didn't steal my wallet!).*

Epilepsy and your rights

The Americans with Disabilities Act (ADA) is a pioneering civil rights law. Patterned on laws that bar discrimination based on race, ethnicity, or gender, the ADA mandates access to all public and most private facilities for disabled citizens. It's usually invoked to make sure people with physical disabilities have access to wheelchair ramps, elevators, grab bars, and other aids to using public or private accommodations. It also prevents handicapped people from most forms of job discrimination by employers, employment agencies, state and local governments, and labor unions.

In schools, the ADA does more than force the district to install handicapped-accessible restrooms and wheelchair ramps for physical access. It mandates that children with disabilities have the right to be involved in all school activities, not just classroom-based educational activities. This includes band, chess club, chorus, sports, camping trips, field trips, and any other activities of interest to your child that are school-sponsored or school-affiliated. If your child will need accommodations or support to take advantage of these activities, you should list this in the Individualized Education Plan (IEP). If you do not have an IEP, a 504 plan can be used. (See Chapter 4 for more information on this topic.)

The ADA prevents day care centers, health clubs, and other privately owned facilities from refusing to admit and serve people with epilepsy. The ADA also protects people with epilepsy against mandatory identification rules: i.e., stores cannot require that check-writers have a valid driver's license, because many people with epilepsy cannot obtain one. A valid state identification card must be an acceptable alternative.

The ADA does not allow prospective employers to ask applicants medical questions, unless an applicant has a visible disability, such as a missing limb, or volunteers information about his medical history. Any questions must be limited to asking the applicant to describe or demonstrate how she would perform essential job functions.

Medical inquiries are allowed after a job offer has been made, or during a pre-employment medical exam.

Employers must provide reasonable accommodations unless they cause undue hardship to the company. An accommodation is a change in duties, work hours, job procedures, equipment, or environment. An employer does not have to make these changes if they would be very costly, disruptive, or unsafe.

Employers may not discriminate because of family illness. For instance, if an employee has a child who has epilepsy, the employer cannot treat the employee differently because she thinks the employee will miss work or file expensive health insurance claims.

Employers are not required to provide health insurance, but if they do, they must offer it fairly to all employees.

The Equal Employment Opportunity Commission (EEOC) enforces the Title 1 (employment) parts of the ADA. Call (800) 669-4000 for enforcement information and (800) 669-3362 for enforcement publications. Other sections are enforced, or have their enforcement coordinated, by the US Department of Justice (Civil Rights Division, Public Access Section). The Justice Department's ADA web site is *http://www.usdoj.gov/crt/ada/adahom1.htm.*

The ADA's Catch-22 clause

One of the ADA's primary authors, former congressman Tony Coelho, is a person with epilepsy. Although protecting persons with seizure disorders was a goal specifically mentioned by Coelho and others during the Congressional debate over the ADA, recent court decisions have limited its use.

Specifically, one decision found that when a person's condition can be "fixed" by a device or medication (in one case, a truck driver whose poor eyesight could be corrected with glasses; in another, a person with high blood pressure controlled by medication), that person is no longer eligible for ADA protection in the workplace. Disability advocates are working furiously to ensure that the ADA is either reinterpreted by the courts or augmented by more specific laws.

One factor that can help you get around this Catch-22 situation is that the medications that control seizures can themselves diminish your ability to work and accomplish activities of daily life. Both seizures and medication use can impair your ability to drive, care for yourself, marry, or have children. If you can document such impairments, you should be considered substantially disabled under the ADA and therefore worthy of its protection.

The disability rights law that preceded the ADA—the Rehabilitation Act of 1973, the same law that created 504 plans for students with special needs—has been interpreted as covering people with epilepsy on many occasions. Until the current ADA problem is fixed, people who experience job discrimination due to seizures may need to invoke this law for protection instead. If you need help with discrimination issues, your state protection and advocacy office offers free assistance to people with disabilities.

What to do about discrimination

If you feel that you have been discriminated against due to your disability or a relative's disability, immediately contact the EEOC, the Canadian Human Rights Commission (CHRC), or your nation's disability rights commission.

In the US, a charge of discrimination generally must be filed within 180 days of when you learned of the discriminatory act. Although you do not need an attorney to file a complaint, a lawyer experienced in job discrimination cases can help you draft the complaint to make it more likely to be successful.

The federal Rehabilitation Act bans public and private employers that receive public funds from discriminating on the basis of disability. The following employees are not covered by the ADA, but are covered by the Rehabilitation Act:

- Employees of the executive branch of the federal government (Section 501 of the Rehabilitation Act)

- Employees of employers who receive federal contracts and have fewer than 15 workers (Section 503 of the Rehabilitation Act)

- Employees of employers who receive federal financial assistance and have fewer than 15 workers (Section 504 of the Rehabilitation Act)

If you are a federal employee (Section 501), you must file a claim within 30 days of the job action against you. If you are an employee whose employer has a federal contract (Section 503), you must file a complaint within 180 days with your local Office of the US Department of Labor, Office of Federal Contract Compliance Programs. If your employer receives federal funds (Section 504), you have up to 180 days to file a complaint with the federal agency that provided funds to your employer, or you can file a lawsuit in a federal court. The federal Rehabilitation Act is enforced by the Civil Rights Division of the Department of Justice, which can be reached at (202) 514-4609. You may choose to call your state Office of Civil Rights first.

In Canada, the Canadian Human Rights Act provides essentially the same rights as the ADA. The act is administered by the Canadian Human Rights Commission. You can get further information by calling the national CHRC office at (613) 995-1151.

In other nations, disability protections may be quite different. All countries in the European Community come under the EC's civil rights laws, and many have more restrictive laws of their own. Your best resource for specific advice is usually a national epilepsy advocacy group.

Seizure disorders and employment

It's a sad truth that many people with seizure disorders are unemployed or underemployed, despite a strong work ethic. Often the problem begins during the teen years, when young people with disabilities may not receive encouragement and opportunities for job training and higher education.

School counselors, and many parents, are not always aware of the options available for people with disabilities in the job market. Their expectations may also be too low, relegating challenged individuals to poorly paid or unreliable work.

Transition planning

Transition planning is the official name for the task of helping teenagers with disabilities get ready for the adult world. It's a process that should begin as early as possible—in fact, for high-schoolers receiving special education services, it's a mandatory part of the Individualized Education Plan (IEP) process.

Transition planning should include vocational testing; career counseling; planning for further education via apprenticeship, trade school, or college; social skills work if needed; and training in areas of daily living that may present a challenge for some people with partial seizures, such as driving, cooking, and managing financial affairs.

Quality transition planning programs involve supervised work experience, job shadowing, and formal mentoring arrangements, helping young people build their resumes and get the contacts they need to find real jobs after high school. They can also involve job coaching services and on-campus programs (such as summer coursework at a college) that prepare students for a successful higher education experience.

Vocational rehabilitation

In the US, every state has a vocational rehabilitation agency that provides services to individuals in the state where they live (not work). The Rehabilitation Act of 1992 requires that state vocational rehabilitation agencies work with schools to provide the help that youth with disabilities need to move from high school to the workplace, so they are often a key part of transition planning programs.

These agencies are also available to adults with disabilities who need help getting trained or retrained for employment.

The federal Rehabilitation Act requires the states to provide the following minimum services:

- Evaluation of potential for rehabilitation.

- Counseling.

- Placement services.

- Physical accommodations. The state does not have to provide equipment, but it does have to help you determine what equipment is needed.

Some states have Vocational Rehabilitation scholarship money that provides an amount comparable to tuition at a state university for vocational training. They may also provide information on private vocational rehabilitation programs in their state, such as training and placement services provided by Goodwill Industries, St. Vincent de Paul, and similar organizations.

To locate your state rehabilitation agency, look in the government pages under Labor, Human Resources, Education, Public Welfare, Human Services, Vocational Rehabilitation Services, or Rehabilitation Services.

If you think that your state is denying you appropriate rehabilitation services, you can file a complaint with the US Department of Education, Rehabilitation Services Administration, Office of the Commissioner, Office of Special Education and Rehabilitation Services, 330 C St. SW, Washington, DC 20202, (202) 732-1282. For information about on-the-job accommodations, contact the Job Accommodation Network at (800) 526-7234 or (800) ADA-WORK.

Off-limits careers

Despite the ADA and other civil rights laws, people who have seizures may find themselves barred from some types of occupations, including military service, flying a plane, driving a train, and hazardous work in which temporary impairment of consciousness or uncontrolled movement could cause injury to oneself or others.

You may hear that epilepsy, or even simply having once taken antiseizure medication, is always a disqualification for military service. This may have been the case at one time, but currently most branches of the US military are willing to consider at least some people with epilepsy. If you have been diagnosed with a form of epilepsy that normally remits in adulthood, you may be able to join the military. If you have active but well-controlled epilepsy and also have a desirable skill to offer, such as computer programming or nursing, recruiters may consider you for certain types of military service.

People with epilepsy usually cannot enter the infantry, flight school, elite commando groups like the Navy SEALs, and other positions where their disability could be dangerous or where wartime conditions could force them to go without needed medications while in the field. All applicants who are granted a medical waiver that allows them to enlist despite a health condition must be able to pass the regular physical and make it through basic training, just like other recruits.

Some people in active military service who are then diagnosed with epilepsy have been given a medical discharge, while others have simply shifted to a specialty where their disability can easily be accommodated. Today's military is usually willing to make a good-faith effort to keep those personnel who want to re-enlist, as training a replacement can be very expensive.

Epilepsy can affect your employability in other fields, depending on the laws and regulations in force where you live. Ken, age 30 and living in Canada, had to change his career plans due to seizures:

> I had psychological counseling for three years, got help from disabled student services workers so I could start college, and haven't looked back since. I graduated from the university in 1996 with a BA in English, with Special Education/Learning Disabilities minor. After being rejected for classroom teaching because of my seizures, I began work in disabled student services, doing research on adaptive technology and student programs.

If your epilepsy begins after you are already in a position where it would normally be contraindicated, the consequences are largely up to your employer. The ADA says that if your disability poses a major inconvenience or danger, your employer can either shift you to another position or, if no such position is available, let you go.

Coping on the job

If a seizure could realistically cause you to harm yourself or others—for example, if you are in charge of running dangerous machinery or driving a vehicle—you must tell your employer or be legally liable for any harm that occurs as a result of not doing so. The financial damages could be substantial, so it's far better to tell a trusted administrator in the workplace and devise an emergency plan.

Some people may need to change jobs or their work conditions because of symptoms they experience. If your seizures are affecting your ability to perform work that you used to be able to do, you are definitely under the ADA's protection and can invoke it when asking for a transfer to a different position or a change in job duties. You can also use it to get accommodations on the job, such as a schedule that prevents sleep deprivation or a change in office lighting. Simply explaining your symptoms, and providing a letter from your physician attesting that they are due to a medical issue, may help your employer understand how seizures can affect your job performance.

Larry, age 33, has found that some after-effects and long-term effects of his partial seizures can be debilitating on the job:

> If I have a lot of seizures, I'm exhausted for most of the day, and I have a very bad headache. Because I'm tired, this often induces further seizure activity. My memory has gone to hell in a handbasket, and I'm very clumsy. My speech, which has always been very good, has now deteriorated quite significantly.

Flexible work arrangements can be great for patients like Larry. That said, many people with partial seizure disorders choose not to inform their employer, either because they feel their episodes do not pose a risk to anyone, or because they fear losing their job if their epilepsy is revealed. If your assessment of potential risk to others is correct, then this is a matter of personal choice.

If you do choose to inform your employer and he feels that no safety issues are involved, you are not under a legal obligation to tell everyone else in the workplace. Most people have found that informed coworkers are more likely to accept unusual behavior that results from seizures if they understand that it has a medical cause, although some people cannot seem to overcome their prejudices.

Medical leave

If you need to be away from work for a while due to worsening symptoms or treatment needs, you may have legal job protection available to you. Since August 1993, the Family and Medical Leave Act (FMLA) has protected US workers in large companies who need a leave of absence. Only employees who work 25 hours per week or more for one year are covered, and only if they work for a company with 50 or more employees within a 75-mile radius.

The Family and Medical Leave Act does the following:

- Provides 12 weeks of unpaid leave during any 12-month period for one's own medical needs or to care for a seriously ill spouse, child, or parent. Sometimes employees can take intermittent leave, which means shortening your normal work schedule.

- Provides 12 weeks of unpaid leave for the birth of a child, or due to placement of a child for adoption or foster care.

- Requires employers to continue benefits, including health insurance, during the leave period.

- Requires employees to attempt to schedule leaves so as not to disrupt the workplace, and to give 30 days' notice if possible.

- Requires employers to put returning employees in the same position or in an equivalent position.

Employers should have procedures in place for medical leaves covered by the FMLA. Usually you will need to present your employer with documentation from your doctor stating why the leave is necessary and how long it is expected to be for.

The FMLA is enforced by the Employment Standards Administration, Wage and Hour Division, US Department of Labor, and the courts. You can find the nearest Wage and Hour Division office in the US government pages of your telephone directory. You have up to two years to file a FMLA complaint or a lawsuit if your employer does not abide by the law.

Seizures and pregnancy

The hormonal changes of pregnancy can increase a woman's risk of seizures, so medication may be necessary for the mother's health even though it does have drawbacks. This is a particular problem for women with a history of eclamptic seizures (seizures during and related to pregnancy). Women who have one or more seizures per month despite treatment are likely to experience an increase in seizures during pregnancy. The reasons for this phenomenon are not yet known, but may include increased estrogen levels, which lower the seizure threshold; hormonal changes that could cause medications to be metabolized differently; nausea and vomiting, which can cause electrolyte imbalances; sleep disturbance; and other factors.[4]

All of the anti-epileptic drugs (AEDs) are believed to be capable of causing birth defects. About 2 percent of all infants are born with some type of birth defect, ranging from negligible differences to life-threatening conditions. Infants born to women who take just one AED run a birth defect risk of about 3 percent, although there is a slightly higher percentage of more severe defects. The most common birth defects attributed to AEDs are heart defects, orofacial clefting (cleft lip or palate and related abnormalities), malformations of the genitals or urinary tract, and neural tube defects like spina bifida.[5]

Taking multiple anti-epilepsy drugs causes the highest risk, especially when the combination used includes both benzodiazepine tranquilizers and other AEDs. Women who take four AEDs run about a 20 percent risk of having an infant with a birth defect.[6] The most serious problems are seen when AEDs, either alone or in combination, are taken during the first three months of pregnancy.

Recent studies indicate that the greatest risk of birth defects from a single AED comes from taking carbamazepine or valproate during the first trimester, and that with valproate that risk increases as the dosage increases. Phenobarbital may not cause a significant risk when used alone, but does when combined with caffeine, whether from caffeinated drinks or from medications that contain caffeine.[7]

Cheri, age 29, discusses the special fears of women who take AEDs:

> We don't have children yet, but this is certainly something we have considered and are continuing to consider. I am on new medications that the medical world is still uncertain about where pregnancy is concerned, so I have been on birth control from the start.

As time progressed, however, it came to our attention through our own research that Tegretol, which I was also taking, decreases the efficacy of contraceptives. It alarmed us that, while each of my doctors was well aware of what the other was prescribing, this detail had not been caught by either of them. They each recognized the problem, of course, when it was brought to their attention. I am now using an IUD.

The majority of women who take AEDs during pregnancy give birth to healthy, normal infants, and much is now known about how to minimize the risk of AED-associated birth defects. All sexually active women of child-bearing age should take a regular multivitamin containing 1 to 5 milligrams of folic acid, whether or not they also take AEDs, to guard against neural tube birth defects like spina bifida.

Many epileptologists, as well as some obstetricians and midwives trained to manage high-risk patients, have experience in assisting women with epilepsy through successful pregnancies. Talk to your doctor about ways to prepare for a planned pregnancy, such as taking a folic acid supplement and adjusting your medications. You may also want to discuss genetic testing at this time, if you have an inheritable seizure disorder.

The current recommendation for AED use during pregnancy is to use the minimum number of medications at the lowest effective dose. You may be able to minimize your AED dose more than usual during pregnancy by making stress-reducing lifestyle changes and trying some alternative therapies like those discussed in Chapter 6 of this book. Don't stop taking your medication suddenly just because you become pregnant; work with your doctor to minimize risk, both to your health and your baby's.

The American College of Obstetricians and Gynecologists has issued an excellent guide to handling seizure disorders during pregnancy, which is listed in Appendix A.

Some AEDs, notably phenytoin, phenobarbital, and carbamazepine, can also interfere with blood clotting, which could be hazardous during childbirth. This problem can be controlled by taking a vitamin K supplement during the last month of pregnancy.

Most AEDs do pass through breast milk, but they are usually well tolerated by breastfeeding infants. However, some babies may become irritable when exposed to these medications. Breastfeeding conveys many health benefits, however, so talk to your doctor or a lactation specialist about handling any problems that may occur during breastfeeding.

Because not all birth defects are immediately visible, it's also important for infants to receive regular follow-up care if they have been exposed to AEDs.

Driving: Law, reality, and reason

Many years ago, this author was riding in the back seat of a car whose driver had a tonic-clonic seizure behind the wheel. Since we were on a winding mountain road, it was a frightening situation. Tragedy was averted, but the incident was a sobering event for one young man with epilepsy, and an example of why all US states and most countries place limits on driving by people with seizure disorders.

Jackie, age 43, tells how she has coped with her inability to drive:

> In 1980 I had my first wreck due to epilepsy. They pulled my license away. I was told I'd have to be seizure-free for one full year to get it back. What?!! I was having worse seizures than I'd ever had in my life. I was living in a small town of 3,000, so small there's not even a taxi service. I thought I'd never adjust. Then I found out the warm, caring nature of small-town folks. I could never have made it without our friends in this town. I had to do without my license for thirteen years as an adult.

Of course, most people can control their seizures reasonably well with medication, and others have consistent auras that let them get off the road before losing consciousness. Many people with partial seizures do not lose consciousness at all, although even alteration of consciousness can make driving unwise. The majority of people with partial seizures retain the ability to drive for all or most of their adult lives, although they may refrain during periods of more severe symptoms.

Only you and your doctor can determine whether and when it's safe for you to drive a car. Most states require between three months and one year of freedom from seizures before you can receive permission to drive. Some require physicians treating people with epilepsy to give their patients' names to the state Department of Motor Vehicles; others rely on patients to be truthful when they apply for a license.

If you can document a seizure-free period of your state's required length, your regular driver's license may be reinstated or reissued with conditions. However, you may be unable to regain or obtain certain types of commercial driver's licenses.

The Epilepsy Foundation maintains a very complete directory of state laws governing driving at *http://www.epilepsyfoundation.org/advocacy/drivelaw/driving.html*. As each state's laws differ and may change over time, read your Department of Motor Vehicles guidelines for getting and keeping a license.

Fear of losing a driver's license and losing freedom of movement as a result is the main reason many people do not tell their doctors about having seizures and miss out on getting treatment. This practice is both unsafe and unwise. If you do not reveal your seizures and have an accident as a result, you can be legally liable for financial and even criminal damages. You also place yourself and others at risk.

If you know in your heart that you should not drive, do the responsible thing and stop. There are alternatives to driving, including taking a taxi or being driven by others, using public transportation, riding a bicycle (if that is safe for you), and walking. You may need to make difficult choices about where you will live, work, shop, and get medical care if your ability to drive will probably be impaired for a long time, but changing your lifestyle is preferable to putting your life at risk.

In the US, special transportation services are available for disabled people who have difficulty using regular public transportation. This can include specially equipped cabs or mini-buses that come to your home. In some cases, these services are paid for by Medicare or Medicaid (usually for medical appointments only); in others, you will need to pay for the service yourself, although its cost may be subsidized. Contact your local transportation authority or disability services office to find out more about your options.

One new option that you may consider if you do drive is installing an emergency alert system in your car, such as the OnStar system, or carrying a cellular phone with an alert feature. This can provide extra peace of mind for you and your family, just in case you need to pull over because of an impending seizure. You can use it to call for emergency help, contact a friend or family member for assistance, or let someone know that you'll be delayed. Some systems also provide assistance with directions and can even help others find you if you're lost, which can be helpful if you experience confusion after a seizure.

Automotive journalist John Matras has an excellent article available online about temporarily losing his license due to adult-onset partial seizures; see "Trouble Afoot" at *http://www.o-c-s.com/epilepsy/jlmatras.htm.*

Leisure activities

Seizures should not prevent anyone from enjoying leisure activities, including sports and swimming. With appropriate precautions, people with epilepsy can take part in almost any sort of physical activity. In fact, pursuing these interests can be very important for strengthening both your self-esteem and your body. Many people with epilepsy feel that regular exercise actually helps to prevent seizures.

People with epilepsy should not swim alone and should inform pool or health club management about how to handle a seizure episode if one occurs in the water or elsewhere in the facility. People whose seizures derive from head injuries can minimize their risk of re-injury by wearing protective headgear, although they should probably avoid hard-contact sports like football or rugby unless their doctor gives permission. If loss of coordination or impairment of consciousness occurs during your seizures, discuss coping strategies with your doctor and a facility manager or coach before you start an exercise or sports regimen.

If fatigue, impaired motor skills, or other effects of your seizures make leisure activities difficult, be sure to explore the possibility of getting physical or occupational therapy. Along with medication changes, these therapies can sometimes open up new possibilities for staying in shape and enjoying a fuller life.

Finding and building support

As the 17th century poet John Donne said, no man is an island. We all need to rely on others to a greater or lesser extent. The word support means different things to different people. For some, it's emotional support that comes to mind first, while for others it denotes practical help in areas like transportation.

Only you can decide what kind of support you and your family need. Often accepting that you need help is difficult, especially for those raised in the American culture of rugged individualism. But it's something that you must do if you don't want a disability to dictate your life choices.

Once you have identified a need that requires outside help, there are many places to look for support. Assistance may come from a friend or family member, someone at work or at your child's school, an epilepsy support group or advocacy organization, a community service agency, religious institution, or government agency. Try to think of several different resources, just in case one doesn't work out.

Ken tells about services in his area of Canada:

> Some support comes from neurological, brain injury, and general social support agencies, but there are not very good support programs specifically designed for people with epilepsy here yet. My work in disabled student services showed me that the stigmas and assumptions about mental deficiency make full development of potential (education and employment) difficult for many people with epilepsy. We are currently in the process of developing workshops that teach how to properly disclose your condition to offer real understanding, independence through social support, and workplace support. I am working specifically with employment agencies, rehabilitation agencies, and special education and counseling workers.

Often your best resource is other people with partial seizure disorders. They've been where you are now as a patient or as a parent and can offer advice based on their own experiences. They may know about community resources you haven't heard of. You can make contact through local epilepsy support groups, a nearby epilepsy treatment center, or online—see Appendix A for a list of possible meeting places on the Internet.

Online support groups like the EPILEPSY-L list (*http://home.ease.lsoft.com/ Archives/Epilepsy-L.html*) are a great option for people in rural areas, those who may have worries about the stigma attached to their condition, and those whose work and family schedules make attending meetings difficult. These discussion groups, which can be accessed either through email alone or via the Web, give you a forum for asking questions and sharing your knowledge with others in need. Participants can be as anonymous as they wish to be. Specific lists may be available for certain types of seizure conditions or people, such as lists for parents of children on the ketogenic diet. You might want to do a search on a web site like eGroups (*http://www. egroups.com*) to see whether a list that meets your needs is available or could be started, or talk to your Internet service provider about list-management options. The Epilepsy Foundation has also begun to sponsor online chat events and "meetings" that may be a valuable resource, especially for newly diagnosed persons.

If you have never felt able to ask for what you needed, or are afraid of becoming dependent on people or services that may not be reliable, you may want to seek out a professional case manager or advocate. This is a person who can investigate your options and secure needed services on your behalf. Anything a case manager or advocate does should be done with your permission and direction, of course. These services may be available through your health plan or from a community services agency. You can also choose to pay a case manager or advocate yourself, if you prefer.

Income support

Most people with epilepsy are financially self-supporting, but for those whose seizures make work impossible, help is available. Although most income support programs are based on having a permanently disabling condition, some are structured to meet short-term needs as well. For example, if you need to have brain surgery, you may be able to access temporary income support during the recovery period.

People with partial seizure disorders can find it difficult to access the federal Social Security Disability Income (SSDI) and Social Security Income (SSI) programs. The regulations as currently written define disabling epilepsy as having more than one major seizure with loss of consciousness and convulsions per month, or having more than one minor motor seizure with alteration or loss of consciousness per week, despite taking prescription anti-epileptic drugs for at least three months. The psychiatric symptoms experienced by some partial seizure disorders (such as difficulty with mood control, extreme fatigue, chronic pain, or thought disturbances) may also be used as qualifying factors.

Kathy, who has had temporal lobe epilepsy since early childhood, decided after many years that she needed income support:

> As an adult, I've found the stigma problem is no different...people are as ignorant as they were when I was in grade school. I can no longer work because of the major ignorance. I had 58 jobs in a thirteen-year span, until I said "no more." I now collect Social Security Disability. I look at the positive side of temporal lobe epilepsy. It doesn't bother me that much—it's society's attitude toward it that has hindered my life, not epilepsy itself.

To apply for these programs, call your local Social Security office. There are benefits options for children with disabilities as well as for adults. Incidentally, eligibility for SSDI or SSI can bring with it Medicaid, which is the federal health insurance plan—a great advantage for those who have not been able to get insurance on the open market or through an employer.

In Europe, Canada, Australia, and New Zealand, disability benefits and financial support for carers are somewhat easier to obtain. Contact your local benefits authority for more specific information, and see Chapter 7, *Healthcare and Insurance*, for additional information.

Today very few options are closed to people with epilepsy, and there are many more tools for battling outdated notions and persevering against the odds. The greatest gift you can give to your child or cultivate within yourself is the confidence that, with information and support, you can surmount this obstacle and reach your goals.

CHAPTER 4

Growing Up with Partial Seizure Disorders

THIS CHAPTER COVERS ISSUES of primary concern to parents: the effect of seizure activity on child development, how to access early intervention and special education services when needed for a child with partial seizure disorders, and how to accommodate special needs in childhood social situations. Parents may also want to consult Chapter 3, *Living with Partial Seizure Disorders*, for ideas that apply to teens as well as adults.

Seizures and development

Mild developmental delays are fairly common in children with epilepsy, as are the minor behavior problems that can be a side effect of slowed development. In most cases, children who are just a few months behind schedule will catch up eventually and will progress quicker if provided with a little extra structure and assistance.

Some children with seizure disorders have more significant developmental delays that are directly related to seizure activity itself. In other cases, developmental delay is another manifestation of the same underlying cause that has produced the seizures, such as brain injury.

All children with seizure disorders should receive regular screening for developmental delays. This is usually a simple matter of talking with the child's pediatrician about whether your child is meeting developmental milestones. The doctor should also check for physical signs of developmental disorders, such as feeding problems or smaller than normal height and weight. If problems are indicated, your doctor can help you choose a course of action.

Sometimes seizure medications are part of the problem. If a medication is sedating your child too much or causes slowed thought processes (cognitive

85

blunting), your child may miss out on normal childhood activities and learning opportunities. He may not have enough energy to practice the movements that eventually lead to walking, for example, leading to weakened muscles. Careful changes to medications can help your child avoid these unwanted side effects while maintaining seizure control.

If your child is falling further and further behind, and especially if he is losing abilities previously gained, it's important to seek an immediate and very thorough developmental and medical evaluation. Moderate to severe developmental delay will not necessarily resolve itself in time, although many pediatricians have been taught that this is the case. Nor is it inevitable and untreatable. Interventions may include medication (or medication changes, as previously noted), special education, occupational or physical therapy, and other techniques that often help to jump-start stalled development in young children.

The outcome is best when developmental issues are met head on and at the earliest possible age. In the US, there are both public and private programs available (as well as therapeutic services such as speech therapy and physical therapy) through school districts, university medical centers, major hospitals, and private practitioners.

In the US, early intervention is the primary name used for a package of services available at no cost to children with disabilities, including developmental delay. These programs provide screening, evaluation, and direct services for infants and pre-school children. Similar programs are available to families in most other countries in the developed world.

Early Intervention (EI) programs can include therapeutic services in the home, a clinic, or a special pre-school. Early Intervention programs can also help families find resources in the community, such as parenting classes, respite care, and support groups. Based on observing and testing your child, the early intervention team will create an Individualized Family Service Plan (IFSP) that lays out what services your child needs, who will provide them, where, and how often.

Gia, mother of 5-year-old James, says:

> It's so important that parents know that early intervention services are available for children—from physical therapy to speech therapy to vision services—regardless of ability to pay in many cases, right from birth up to preschool age (when most public schools take over). In most

states, a parent's, daycare worker's, or pediatrician's request can get an evaluation from a local developmental services or early intervention agency.

In our case, an astute daycare worker was concerned that our young toddler was not progressing as he should with hand/eye coordination (he kept missing his mouth with a spoon). This led to an evaluation by our local agency, and soon we had physical therapy services in place. Later on, it was learned that his underlying condition was an optic glioma [a type of tumor], which had caused peripheral vision loss. In no time at all, his early intervention services were expanded to include orientation and mobility/vision services as well as speech therapy, which he needed following brain surgery.

We think one of the reasons that our son has done so well and is on-track now at age 5 is due to all the intervention that was possible from an early age.

To find the nearest early intervention program, call your school district. Most of these programs are offered through the schools, although some programs for children from birth to three may be provided through a state health department, regional center, or other government agency.

Schools and special education

Before your child enters kindergarten or first grade, contact your local school district to find out about special education services. Most children with epilepsy, including those who have tonic-clonic seizures, do not need to be in special classrooms or have a certain type of educational program. They can attend the same classes in the same neighborhood school as their peers without disabilities. However, parents must communicate with their child's school about the diagnosis. The potential stigma of labeling a child as having epilepsy is far less serious than what will happen if the school labels the same child as a behavior problem or a lazy student who refuses to do his work. Parents can also use the special education laws to put supports into place for children who may have seizures at school, and to ensure that teachers, counselors, and administrators are well-educated about potential health concerns.

Of course, some children who have seizures also have developmental delays, learning disabilities, or additional psychiatric, behavioral, or mobility problems. All of these conditions deserve special attention and assistance at school.

Theresa is the mother of 14-year-old Bryce, who began having partial complex seizures after a complication of chemotherapy for childhood leukemia caused a stroke-like event:

> We have lots of developmental and educational concerns. We don't know if it's from seizures or the chemo, but he has definite cognitive problems and his short-term memory is impaired, and with that comes some socialization difficulties.
>
> As for school, how it goes depends on how hard you want to work at it. It has been a process for me. You learn to be pretty pushy, and you have to stay on top of it all the time. I bet I've already gone to four meetings this year just trying to set up his program for high school. He has an aide at this time for his safety, and so he can learn. I go to the people who work with him directly if I feel the need to.

Federal law specifically mandates that all children receive a free and appropriate education (referred to in special education circles as a "FAPE"), regardless of disability. That means providing, free of charge, special education programs, speech therapy, occupational therapy, physical therapy, psychiatric services, and other interventions that can help the child learn.

Several laws protect your child's access to an education. These include Section 504 of the Rehabilitation Act of 1973, the Individuals with Disabilities Education Act (IDEA), the Americans with Disabilities Act (ADA), and other state and federal laws concerning disability rights and special education.

504 plans

At the very least, all children with a seizure disorder should be covered by what's called a 504 plan—an agreement between the child's family and the school about accommodations that can help him attend school successfully. This name comes from Section 504 of the Rehabilitation Act of 1973, one of the very first laws mandating educational help for students with disabilities, which lays out the regulations for such plans. A 504 plan can be written mostly by a team made up of the parents and teachers or school administration, with minimal involvement by the school district's administrators.

Unlike special education eligibility, Section 504 eligibility is not based on having a certain type of disability. Instead, it is based on having a physical or mental impairment that substantially limits a major life activity, such as learning. Note that in contrast to IDEA regulations, learning is not the only activity that applies: 504 plans can cover other major life activities, such as breathing, walking, and socialization. Children are also covered by this law if they simply have a record (such as a medical diagnosis) of such an impairment or are regarded as having such an impairment.

A 504 plan is a good idea even if your child has never had an academic or behavior problem in school. The nature of partial seizure disorders dictates that new symptoms could emerge at any time and have unexpected effects on school performance. Your child's 504 plan can put procedures into place regarding who will give out medication and where it will be stored, communication between home and school, the use of certain organization systems for homework and books, exemption from timed tests, or what to do if your child has a seizure at school, just to give a few examples. It can include procedures for giving emergency medication, calling for outside help, and keeping the child and others safe until that help arrives. Without advance planning, it's easy for a bad day to turn into a crisis.

Having a plan in place to deal with seizures at school is important, whether it's a 504 plan or part of an IEP. Lucy tells how her school handles her son Harry's partial seizures:

> If he feels the aura, he alerts a teacher and they let him lie down
> briefly in the nurse's office or in a teacher conference room. Only on really
> bad days does the school nurse call me and suggest that I come get him.
> The other kids are pretty understanding, as they know he will come out of
> it within a few minutes. It can be frightening to watch for the first time,
> but once you get used to the pattern, you simply teach around it, recog-
> nizing that he probably lost whatever you taught him in the few minutes
> just before the episode.

If you apply for 504 status and are still denied services, appeal this decision to your school district's 504 compliance officer. If that doesn't produce results, contact your state's office of civil rights. Even students with mild ADHD or occasional asthma attacks qualify for assistance under a 504 plan.

Some special education advocates recommend that parents request a 504 evaluation at the same time they start the process of special education evaluation. It may confuse your district because it isn't a common practice, but it will save time in obtaining some services and accommodations if services are denied under IDEA and you have to appeal.

Because most 504 plans are fairly uncomplicated documents, you may be tempted to simply set up an informal agreement with your child's school instead. Don't do it. Informal agreements only work as long as the people involved stay the same, and as long as everyone chooses to honor them. If your school gets a new principal or your child's teacher decides to change plans in midstream, you'll be right back where you started. With a 504 plan, you have a document that mandates access to needed services. If your school or district decides not to follow it, you can appeal directly to your district's 504 compliance officer and/or your state office of civil rights.

Special education and IDEA

Special education has been revolutionized by IDEA, a set of comprehensive rules and regulations that was most recently revised and expanded in 1997. IDEA's mission is to ensure that all children get an adequate education, regardless of disabilities or special needs.

The special education process starts with evaluation. In most areas, eligibility is determined by a committee of specialists and teachers, which may be called the eligibility committee, multidisciplinary team (M-team), child study team, or a similar name. As the parent, you should have input during this eligibility process. You will be asked to fill out forms, and you can also request a personal interview with the team and submit information, such as medical evaluations, to help it make a decision.

The eligibility committee will decide if your child has a condition that qualifies him for special education services. Exact language differs between states, but typical qualifying categories include:

- Autistic
- Hearing impaired (deafness)
- Visually impaired
- Both hearing impaired and visually impaired (deaf-blindness)
- Speech and language impaired

- Mentally retarded/developmentally delayed
- Multihandicapped
- Severely orthopedically impaired
- Other health impaired (OHI)
- Seriously emotionally disturbed (SED)
- Severely and profoundly disabled
- Suffering from specific learning disability
- Suffering from traumatic brain injury

Check your state's special education regulations for the list of labels used in your state.

Most children and teens with partial seizure disorders who receive special education services are classified under the OHI label. Those whose seizures primarily affect mood and perception may also qualify under the SED designation, which is often required to access day treatment or residential slots. On the other hand, the SED label may prevent your child from being admitted to some alternative school programs without a fight.

Lucy, mother of 10-year-old Harry, found that the evaluation process was stymied by medical indecision:

> The school was very cooperative after the initial head injury, as the symptoms of postconcussion syndrome were quite evident. The partial seizures began after a second seemingly minor blow to the head...and the school's reaction this time was more mixed. The neurologist said "partial seizures" right away, and the school was sympathetic. But then the neurologist changed his mind, as one EEG was abnormal and another one was normal. The teachers and school nurse then thought he was faking.

> Over the next few months another neurologist also said "no seizures," then "seizures," then "no seizures" again. By this time, however, the teachers and school nurse had witnessed enough episodes that the neurological confusion didn't bother them so much. It was apparent that the child was experiencing something that was causing dilated eyes and significant movement, followed by extreme fatigue, confusion, and loss of memory. It didn't matter so much what it was called...it was interfering with school and homework.

The condition that causes the most impairment in school-related activities will usually be called the primary handicapping condition, and any others that co-exist with it will be called secondary handicapping conditions. For example, a child with partial seizures and dyslexia might be qualified for special education under the primary condition OHI, with specific learning disability as a secondary label.

Although the eligibility committee will take your child's medical diagnosis and the opinions of Early Intervention evaluators into account when they make their determination, qualifying categories are defined by each school district or state department of education in terms of education, not medicine. If your child has an epilepsy diagnosis from a psychiatrist, neurologist, or other physician, the committee can still decide that your child does not meet the educational definition of OHI or another label. This means that either the committee feels your child does not need special services to take advantage of educational opportunities, or that the committee is unwilling to offer your child needed services. Technically, a medical diagnosis of epilepsy should automatically qualify a child for the label OHI, even if his illness is currently controlled via medication or his symptoms are not prominent.

You have the right to appeal the eligibility team's decision about your child's educational label or any other issue. If its decision prevents your child from receiving special education eligibility or needed services, you should do so. It is helpful to prepare a detailed list of ways your child's problems impact his ability to be educated without the added help of special education services.

The Individualized Education Plan (IEP)

When completed, your child's special education evaluation will be the basis of a document that'll soon become your close companion: your child's Individualized Education Plan (IEP). The IEP describes your child's strengths and weaknesses, sets educational goals and objectives for her, and details how these can be met within the context of the school system. Unlike the IFSP used in Early Intervention programs for pre-school children, the IEP is almost entirely about what will happen within school walls. Unless the IEP team agrees to include it, there will be little information about services from outside programs or services provided by or to parents.

The IEP is created during one or more meetings of your child's IEP team, which has a minimum of three members: a teacher, a parent, and a representative from the school district. The district may send more than one representative, and parents may (at their child's peril) choose not to attend. If your child has more than one teacher, or if direct service providers such as an occupational therapist would like to attend, they can all be present. If it is your child's first IEP and first assessment, one team member is required by federal law to have experience with and knowledge of the child's suspected or known disabilities.

Both parents should participate in the IEP process if possible, even if they do not live together. Parents can also bring anyone else they would like: a relative or friend, an after-school caretaker, a health advocate, or a lawyer, for example. This person may act as an outside expert or may simply offer moral support or take notes so that you can participate more freely. The child himself can also be at the IEP meeting if the parents would like—however, it's a good idea to bring a sitter with a young child to avoid disruptions. You want to be able to give the IEP process your full attention, and that's hard if you're also trying to keep a child out of trouble. Most young children find IEP meetings rather boring.

Older teens and self-advocacy

Districts are trying to involve middle school and high school students in the IEP process more often, and this is probably a good trend. Discuss the meeting with your older child and elicit her suggestions in advance. Some adolescents prefer to write up their suggestions rather than (or in addition to) attending the meeting. As with young children, bring someone to take care of your child if she tends to be disruptive, and bring a book or game in case the meeting gets boring. It's not beneficial to force an unwilling child to take part in the meeting.

Recently, parents of older teens in special education have reported a disturbing new trend: school districts that try to circumvent IDEA by making teens "self-advocates" at the age of 18, regardless of their ability to make wise choices, and regardless of their parents' wishes. If—and only if—parents agree, any child in special education who has reached age 18 can take full control of all further contacts with the school district. Needless to say, this is often a very unwise thing to agree to. In most cases, the outcome has been that the child immediately leaves school and loses all services.

If your district tries this ploy, there is a way back in. As an adult self-advocate, your child can appoint another person to advocate for her. That person can be you or, if you prefer, a professional advocate.

Remember that, unless you permit them to end earlier, special education services continue until at least the age of 21, or until the attainment of a regular high school diploma (not a GED or IEP diploma).

Building an IEP

Usually the IEP meeting is held at a school or a district office. However, you can request another location for the meeting if it is necessary—for example, if your child is on homebound instruction or has severe seizures that make caring for him impossible away from the controlled environment of home at this time. The meeting date and time must be convenient to you (and, of course, to the other team members).

Your first IEP meeting should begin with a presentation of your child's strengths and weaknesses. This may be merely a form listing test scores and milestones, or it can include verbal reports of observations by team members—including you. You can use this time to tell the team a little more about your child, her likes and dislikes, her abilities, and the worries that have brought you all together for this meeting. Even if you're repeating information that the team members already know, this kind of storytelling helps other team members see your child as a person rather than just another case.

The IEP itself has two important parts: the cover sheet, usually called the accommodations page, and the goals and objectives pages. Your district may have its own bureaucratic names for these pages, such as a G3 or an eval sheet. If team members start throwing around terms you don't understand, be sure to speak up! If the wrong forms are filled out, or if important paperwork is left undone, you may not have an acceptable IEP at the end of the meeting.

The cover page should summarize any services your child will receive, including who will deliver them, where they will be delivered, and how frequently they will be delivered. It will list the people who participated in creating the IEP, and it may list the names of direct service providers.

Accommodations

The cover page may be combined with or followed by one or more accommodations pages. These should not already be filled out when the IEP meeting begins, as your child's individual goals and objectives should dictate what accommodations will be needed. Partial seizures can affect a child's ability to pay attention and absorb material being taught. Changes in depth perception and other effects can make common classroom activities, such as writing or using scissors, more difficult. Not only can seizures themselves be distracting or confusing, but medications used to control seizures can sometimes cause sleepiness or "brain fog" that gets in the way of learning. As with any chronic health condition, living with epilepsy can also affect a child's self-perception and self-esteem.

Since kids aren't always forthcoming about their symptoms, you may have to ask lots of questions before you get to the root of academic or behavior problems. Teachers and parents should first closely observe the child's academic performance or behavior, and then brainstorm several possible solutions with the child and her teachers. You may have to try a few before finding a workable accommodation. Often the child already knows some strategies that work and simply needs your approval to put them in place.

Lucy says her son's seizures have an effect on his school performance, but it's different from what teachers sometimes expect:

> One thing I've noticed about the schools—every time you meet a new teacher and need to explain that your son has seizures, they instantly think of grand mal seizures. They are fearful he will fall and hurt himself or someone else. Yet he doesn't lose consciousness during these episodes. He may be confused and disoriented, but he isn't any more likely to fall than any other child. He even swims on a competitive swim team! Stereotypes die hard.

Programs designed to meet an individual student's needs must be flexible due to the waxing and waning nature of seizure disorders. Students with epilepsy may have long periods during which their symptoms are minimal. Teachers can take advantage of these periods to help them make up missed assignments or move ahead rapidly, leaving room to relax a bit during periods when symptoms are more severe. Accommodations no longer needed can be suspended until symptoms flare up again.

Like students with ADD/ADHD, kids with partial seizure disorders can almost always benefit from specific instruction in study and schoolwork skills, including systems for conceiving and completing intensive projects such as essays, reports, and science projects. Successful strategies used by some students include breaking up large projects into small, manageable tasks, each with its own deadline; learning formulas that, if followed, will always turn out a serviceable essay or report; using an assignment or agenda book that teachers and parents check each day; using visual organizing systems, such as color-coded folders or sticky notes, to keep assignments organized and on time; and setting a specific amount of time aside daily for schoolwork. Of course, parents should provide a good environment for studying at home and ensure that extracurricular activities, medical appointments, and family activities do not disrupt a child's regular study sessions.

District representatives tend to see their role in the IEP meeting as being the gatekeeper. They may interpret this as spending as little money as possible or ensuring that children are matched with services that meet their needs, depending on the person, the district, and the situation. Most struggle to balance these goals for the benefit of each child and the district's resources. As your child's advocate, your job is to persuade the representative to tip the scales in your child's favor.

Accommodations that your child may need could include the following:

- A specific type of classroom.

- Provision of other types of environments, such as a resource room setting for certain subjects, mainstreaming for other subjects, or an area for time-outs or self-calming.

- A set procedure for allowing the child to take a self time-out when seizure symptoms begin. For example, your child might quietly show a green card to the teacher, who could send him on his way to the school nurse's office with a nod of her head.

- Class schedules adapted to the child's ability to concentrate and stay alert, especially during times of acute stress (such as just after release from the hospital) and during medication changes.

- Specific learning materials or methods.

- Accommodations for testing, such as untimed tests, extended test-taking times, exemption from certain types of tests, or oral exams (this is an especially good idea for those students who have hand tremor due to medication).

- Permission to use a tape recorder to record lectures and class discussions.

- Permission to share notes with another student or to receive pre-written notes from the instructor.

- Grade arrangements that take into account assignments and school days missed due to symptoms or to hospitalization. These might include estimating semester grades based only on the work that was completed; offering the option of an incomplete grade to allow the student to finish the course when well; or basing grades on some combination of class participation when present, work completed, and a special oral exam.

- A reduced number of required courses for graduation.

- A personal educational assistant, aide, or "shadow"—either a monitoring aide who simply helps with behavior control, or an inclusion or instructional aide.

- Other classroom equipment needed to help your child learn if he has auditory processing or learning disabilities, such as a microphone or sound field system, a slanted work surface, or pencils with an orthopedic grip.

- Preparation and implementation of a behavior plan.

The last item on that list is of particular importance for children with temporal lobe epilepsy, some of whom have episodes of aggressive, self-injurious, or even violent behavior. Children who experience these difficulties, even if behavior problems have so far occurred only at home, should always have a behavior plan in place at school that can be followed in case of an incident. This plan should be written into the IEP. As part of the behavior plan, parents can also let teachers know about any triggers and warning signs that they have discovered, helping them to intervene early and prevent problems when possible.

Goals and objectives

Parents tend to focus on the goals and objectives pages, which usually make up the bulk of the IEP, and often overlook the accommodations pages. That's a mistake. The goals and objectives are all about what your child will do, and if they are not accomplished, no one but your child can be truly held accountable. The accommodations page, however, is about what the school district will do to help make your child able to meet those goals: what services it will provide or pay for, what kind of classroom setting your child will be in, and any other special education help that the district promises to provide.

The accommodations page is where the district's promises are made, so watch out: saying that your child will do something costs the district nothing, but promising that the district will do something has a price tag attached. Be prepared to hear phrases like "I don't want to commit the district to that" over and over, and be prepared to methodically show that the accommodations you're asking for are the only way to meet the goals and objectives the team wants to set.

Nevertheless, it is important to have clear goals and objectives in the IEP, as they help provide direction for your child's education program and give you benchmarks to measure her progress against. You may choose to meet one-on-one with your child's teacher to talk over IEP goals before the big meeting.

Goals should also be written in a way that allows progress to be measured. For example, "Stacey will learn how to use a daily agenda book and new note-taking procedures to help her stay on-task in her schoolwork" is a much more specific and demonstrable goal than "Stacey will learn to be more organized at school." When Stacey's IEP review comes around, her parents can see the agenda book and her notes, ask her teachers how the new procedure was taught, and make sure the goal has been met.

Generally speaking, children in special education programs should be educated to the same standards as all other students whenever that is possible. They should work with the same curriculum and objectives, although specific requirements can be adjusted to fit the child. For example, if third graders in your district are normally required to present a ten-minute oral report about state history, a child with medication-induced fatigue might be allowed to present a shorter oral report, present her report in two parts, or have her written report read out loud by a helper.

As a parent, you'll want to talk to your child's teacher about the academic curriculum in use in your child's school and in the district itself. Make sure that your child is being instructed in the skills, concepts, and facts needed to proceed in school. If you live in one of the many states that are introducing competency standards for all students, make sure that your child (and all children in special education) are not exempted from the same expectations. If your state has set the goal of having all children reading at grade level by fifth grade, for example, your child should be held to the same standard— and offered the special education assistance she may need to achieve it.

High school students' IEPs must also include transition plans to prepare them for college, trade school, or vocational opportunities after high school.

See Chapter 3 for more information on vocational rehabilitation, one of the post–high school options open to some students with seizure disorders.

Children with epilepsy come in all types, from slow to average to gifted. A good IEP doesn't dumb down classes or take away the joy of achieving something difficult; it just ensures that a child with disabilities gets an equal shot. The IEP can provide flexibility while still maintaining appropriate academic standards: for example, permitting your child to audit some courses before taking them for credit, and arranging in advance for using correspondence courses, distance learning (courses taken over the Internet), or independent study to fill in gaps created by hospitalization or periods of more severe symptoms.

Signing the IEP...or not

When the IEP is complete, the accommodations page will include a list of each promise, information about where and when it will be met, and the name of the person responsible for delivering or ensuring delivery. If the complete IEP is acceptable to everyone present, this is probably also where all team members will sign on the dotted line.

You do not have to sign the IEP if it is not acceptable. This fact can't be emphasized enough! If the meeting has ended and you don't feel comfortable with the IEP as it is, you have the right to take home the current document and think about it (or discuss it with your spouse or an advocate) before you sign. You also have the right to set another IEP meeting, and another, and another, until it is truly complete. Don't hinder the process unnecessarily, of course, but also don't let yourself be steamrolled by the district. The IEP is about your child's needs, not the district's needs.

Needless to say, you should never sign a blank or unfinished IEP—it's a bit like signing a blank check. Certain school districts ask IEP meeting participants to sign an approval sheet before even talking about the IEP. Others are in the habit of taking notes for a prospective IEP and asking parents to sign an approval form at the end of the meeting, even though the goals, objectives, and accommodations have not been entered on an actual IEP form. This is not okay. If they insist that you sign a piece of paper, make sure to add next to your name that you are signing because you were present, but that you have not agreed to a final document.

If your child already has an IEP in place from the previous year, this IEP will stay in place until the new one is finalized and signed. If your child does not, you may need to come to a partial agreement with the district while a final IEP is worked out.

If the IEP process becomes contentious, be sure to bring an advocate to the next meeting. A good advocate can help smooth out the bumps in the IEP process while preserving your child's access to a free and appropriate education.

Placement decisions

Today, most special education students receive help in a regular classroom, not a classroom with only disabled children or a special school. Each child with partial seizures is unique, so there's no single school program that has proven successful with all such children.

Two factors govern the choice of school for your child: the most appropriate educational program and the least restrictive environment (LRE). For most children, the least restrictive environment is their neighborhood school, or one very much like it that happens to have an especially good teacher or support services. This is called inclusion, full integration, or mainstreaming.

Full inclusion is not a magical solution to school problems. Too often schools use it to deny special education services to the students who need them. That's why many classroom teachers dread having children with mental or physical disabilities in their classes. Without help from classroom aides and specialists, administrative support, well-written IEPs, and the resources to help each child meet his goals, the teacher's job becomes a nightmare. Parents are often the key to making sure their children are properly served in an inclusive setting. Teachers love parents who go to bat with the administration or district to get needed classroom help.

Perhaps the best advice that successful students with seizure disorders and their parents can offer is that the people and atmosphere of a school count the most, and that one program does not fit all. Some students desire the anonymity and lower social pressure of large public schools, while others thrive in small classes with lots of personal attention. The best school environment is very much an individual thing.

Special classrooms

Some children will not be able to handle the noise, confusion, and demands of a traditional school program. Some troubled schools are, in turn, barely capable of meeting the needs of average students, much less those with special needs. There should be a range of placements available, including staying in the neighborhood school in a mainstream class, spending part or all of the day in a resource room or special education classroom, learning at home with one-on-one instruction, and day treatment or residential placement.

Some children will only need a special classroom for part of the day. Perhaps they need special help with math or reading. A resource room can be part of the solution. This is a space in the school where a special education teacher can help kids meet their individual needs.

Becky, mother of 15-year-old Karl, explains how he uses the school's resource room:

> My son always struggled in school, with difficulties in comprehension, language arts, writing skills, etc. He had his first seizure (complex partial) when he was 11, and the MRI showed a focal point in the right temporal lobe. To me, it all seemed to fit together, and I have no doubt that his learning difficulties are related to seizures. Unfortunately, the meds he is taking, Depakote and Tegretol, seem to make him even more "out of it." All this added with teenage hormones… it is hard to tell what is causing what anymore.
>
> Anyway, he is now in high school, receiving resource help for English and hanging in there. We and the school still need to spend a lot of time with him, making sure school work is done correctly, helping him study for tests, etc.

For those students who do need a full-day special education program, there are many types of self-contained special classrooms. Children with partial seizure disorders are most likely to be sent to a behavioral classroom, where their classmates will be other children whose disabilities impact behavior. In most school districts, behavioral classes are seen as a short-term placement—like a boot-camp class for kids who behave badly. For children whose seizures are not well-controlled or who have developmental delay, this view is neither realistic nor wise. If a particular behavioral class is working well for your child, see what you can do to hold onto that placement.

Most districts have special classes for children with moderate to severe developmental delays (mental retardation, autism, etc.). In small districts, this may be the only special education classroom available. Such a placement might seem like a terrible idea for your child—and it might well be a mistake. However, if the classroom happens to have a very good teacher and will make other needed supports available to your child, it could be worth considering. There may be a stigma attached for your child, of course...especially if the class is in his neighborhood school and his friends will know that he has been put in the "retarded kids class." Many of these classes are actually quite good, with a caring and individualized approach that some of the behavioral classes would do well to emulate. For some kids with partial seizure disorders, especially the very youngest students, there will be times that being the "smart kid" in a developmental delay class is a great solution to a difficult education problem.

Alternative schools

For some students with partial seizure disorders, alternative schools (including charter schools) offer the best mix of high academic expectations, strong behavioral supports, and flexibility. Large urban districts may offer all sorts of public alternative schools, ranging from special schools for at-risk/gang-affected youth, to arts magnet schools. Small, rural districts may have no choices at all. Suburban areas may have only alternative schools that emphasize behavior modification rather than academics, and they often use them as a dumping ground for problem students with little regard for these children's actual needs or abilities.

If your district does offer alternative programs, look before you leap. Visit the site with your child, and ask for a guided tour. Sit in on typical classes. If you can, talk to other parents whose children attend the school, and meet the actual teachers that your child would be working with. Make sure you feel comfortable with the alternative school's philosophy, methods, and objectives. If your child has had difficulty handling school in the past, you don't want to set him up for additional failure by making a hasty decision. Finding the right fit will make school success more likely.

Alternative schools, and in most cases charter schools, will still need to abide by your child's IEP. Often these schools are much more flexible, but occasionally they have been set up with a very specific program in mind, such as a levels-based behavior modification system or an arts-centered program designed for self-directed learners. If you sense that the alternative school is rigid in its format, make sure that format is already a good fit for your child. Like a regular public school that has a one-size-fits-all mentality, alternative schools with a specific mission are unlikely to change their approach, even to meet your child's IEP objectives.

Diagnostic classroom

If your child's diagnosis is still not set in stone, your district might suggest placement in a diagnostic classroom. This classroom might be a joint project of the school district and a regional medical center or medical school, and it is used for long-term medical or psychiatric observation and evaluation of children whose behavior and abilities don't seem to fit the typical profile of one condition. This is not a permanent placement, but if your child's case is especially unusual, she may stay in the diagnostic classroom for quite some time.

A well-run diagnostic classroom offers your family a unique opportunity to have your child seen at length by experts and to try new medications, therapies, and other treatments in a medically savvy setting. Make sure that the classroom staff and doctors involve your whole family in the diagnostic and treatment process. Parents report that some diagnostic classrooms are so patient-centered that they forget to talk to parents after the initial interview process.

Special schools

If your child is unable to attend a regular school, either in an inclusive situation or in a special education classroom, she may be able to go to a special school. If it's public, it will be very much like going to alternative school. Many districts also contract with private schools that work with certain types of students, such as a private school that uses the Orton-Gillingham method to teach students with dyslexia.

Some private schools serve emotionally troubled youth, and a few have a history of working with children whose primary diagnosis is a seizure disorder. Some are excellent, and some are not.

Day treatment centers are a specific type of special school for children with very difficult behaviors, such as self-injurious or aggressive behavior, that make even a self-contained special education classroom inappropriate. They may be attached to or affiliated with a residential school or hospital. At the end of the school day, children in day treatment go home to their families. Good day treatment centers provide medical and psychiatric support, specially trained staff, a very secure environment, and intensive intervention. However, many specialize in the treatment of behavior disorders (such as behavior problems that occur as a result of child abuse) and may not have a full understanding of seizure disorders.

The other problem with many current day treatment programs is that they tend to be conceived as short-term interventions. Slots may be limited to one school year, or even to as little as three months. Students cycle in and out, and staff turnover may also be high. Your child may be in class with children whose behaviors are even more unmanageable than her own.

Residential schools

In some cases, residential programs are your only option. If you live in a small, rural school district, there may simply be no appropriate placement available—assuming that homebound instruction would not be appropriate for your child or your family situation. However, medical need is the most common reason for a child with epilepsy to be in a residential school.

Residential schools offer educational programming and 24-hour care for the child. If your school district asks to send your child to a residential program, the district will pay her tuition and all associated costs. Of course, you also have the option to choose a residential program for your child and pay for it yourself, if you have the financial means.

The best residential programs have staff with a strong medical background, a high level of employee retention, and a commitment to communicating with and working with students' families. As with any other type of school program, you should visit the campus, observe a classroom, see the living quarters, talk to staff and (if possible) students, and try to talk to other parents whose children have attended the school. No place is perfect, but some residential schools have deservedly bad reputations.

Be sure that the school and its staff are able to meet your child's medical needs, including accommodating special diets, managing medications and medical devices, and obtaining on-site emergency help as needed.

Hospital-based education

If your child needs to be an in-patient in a hospital for more than a week or so, you'll need to ensure that his education is continued. If your child is going to have a planned hospitalization, contact the hospital program and find out who's in charge of communicating with patients' schools. There should be a formal school-hospital liaison. Make sure this person is in contact with your child's teacher (or, in the case of a high school student who has many teachers, a homeroom teacher, school counselor, or other person who can act as a go-between) before your child's scheduled entry date and that he has set up an educational program in advance. This might include providing lesson plans and reading lists, sending your child's homework assignments to the hospital, and returning graded papers to you, for example.

If the hospitalization is sudden, you will probably need to act as the go-between yourself. Call your child's teacher or teachers and make arrangements for what they feel would be appropriate work to complete during her stay. Before her release, make plans for what she should do at home while she recuperates, and plan how to make her school reentry successful. You can then make arrangements with hospital staff to ensure that she has the tools and time she needs to do the work. Staff can also let you know if the teacher's plans are too ambitious, and they can provide medical documentation for reducing or even eliminating schoolwork for a while if needed.

Homebound instruction

Homebound instruction is considered the most restrictive school environment, because it involves assigning a teacher to work with your child individually. However, children may prefer homebound instruction to attending a special school or entering a residential program, because it keeps them home with their parents and siblings, even though it does restrict their ability to interact with same-age peers.

Homebound instruction can be delivered by a teacher who comes to your home or another location (such as a public library), via correspondence courses or distance learning arrangements, or with any combination of methods.

If your child is in high school, you'll probably need to make sure his homebound program will help him meet the requirements for graduation. This may mean having the instructor follow specific lesson plans, use certain text-books, or help your child complete required projects.

You'll also want to meet with the homebound instructor privately to explain your child's symptoms, go over her IEP, and talk about grading arrangements.

Homeschooling

In most US states, it is legal for parents to educate their children at home. Each state has its own regulations involving testing, qualifications required of parents, and registration with the state. Homeschooling styles vary as much as parents do, from free-form "unschooling" to home use of purchased curriculum materials.

If you do homeschool, decide in advance whether your child will be working toward a high school diploma (this is possible if you use certain homeschool curricula), a GED, or a portfolio of work. Experienced homeschooling parents can help you consider your options, and can be contacted through local groups or online. Some homeschooling groups have a religious focus and can be contacted through local churches; others can be found through the classified ads of magazines like *Mothering*.

Eligible homeschooled children are entitled to early intervention and special education services. These services may be delivered in the child's home, at a neutral site, or in a nearby school or clinic. This means you can homeschool and still have an IEP with the school district to provide your child with speech therapy, counseling, and other needed services.

It's important to set up socialization opportunities if you are homeschooling. Many homeschooling families share teaching duties with other parents, bringing several children together for certain lessons or activities. Home-schoolers can also choose to take part in extracurricular activities at their neighborhood public school and may even be able to take some classes at school (advanced math, for example) while doing the bulk of their school-work at home.

If you are forced to homeschool your child because your district cannot or will not provide a free and appropriate education program, you may be eligible to be paid to teach your child. This option has worked for parents in very rural areas, as well as for some in districts that could not provide a safe setting for a child with assaultive behaviors or special medical needs.

Private schools

Sometimes parents opt for private school placement directly, at their own cost. Perhaps daily religious instruction is very important to you, or your child's siblings already attend a private school. Luckily, choosing a private school does not automatically disqualify your child from publicly funded early intervention and special education services. To receive public special education services, a child in private school must first be evaluated and qualified within the public system. The IFSP or IEP will determine which services will be delivered, where they will be delivered, and by whom.

In a few areas, parents may be able to use school vouchers to lower the cost of private schools, making this educational option more accessible. Depending on local regulations (and on the mood of the courts), your choices may include parochial schools.

When looking at private school programs, give them the same level of scrutiny to which you would subject a public program. Educational programming for children with partial seizure disorders requires a certain level of knowledge and flexibility that not all schools have, public or private. You can advocate until you're blue in the face, but in the end, private schools do not have to work with your child.

Private schools that accept any form of public funding may be subject to additional regulations. Most are also subject to the Americans with Disabilities Act, which may prevent a school from discriminating against your child due to his disability. However, unlike Section 504 and IDEA, it will not give you tools to require the school to do anything specific to help him learn.

Let the setting fit the child

In between the placement options presented in this chapter are combination settings created to meet a student's specific needs. For example, one student might be able to handle a half-day inclusion program in the morning, then have home-based instruction for other subjects in the afternoon. Another child might be placed in a special class for everything but art and music.

The setting(s) listed in your child's IEP should be reviewed every year (or more often, if you request it) to ensure that the educational program is still meeting his needs and that he is still in the least restrictive setting. It's important to remember that because your child's symptoms may wax and wane drastically, a school setting that once worked well may not work forever.

Monitoring school progress

You can't rely totally on the school or the school district to monitor your child's progress or to ensure compliance with his IEP. Keep a copy of this document and other important notes on hand, and check them against any communications notebooks, progress reports, report cards, and assignments that come home from the school.

Of course you'll want to attend all official meetings, but make a point of just dropping by occasionally on the pretext of bringing your child her coat or having paperwork due at the school office. If you can volunteer an hour a week or so in the school (not necessarily in your child's classroom), that's even better.

If the school is not complying with the IEP, start by talking to the teacher, and work your way up. Most compliance problems can be addressed at the classroom level.

Monitoring the delivery of pull-out services, such as occupational therapy, is one area that can be especially difficult. It seems like a relatively simple task, but parents across the country report that their school district refuses to provide any type of checklist that lets parents see if their child is receiving the services listed in the IEP.

If your IEP includes academic goals, see if there are standardized ways to monitor progress—grades alone aren't always enough. Too often parents are told that their child is participating well and learning, and then they discover that he has not gained new skills or has regressed when an objective measure is used. Ask that your child be tested every year if possible. You are entitled to the results of any standardized tests your child may take. Check the scores to make sure your child is progressing.

Many parents have found that their children are actually regressing due to inadequate classroom support or curriculum. Lack of progress or regression gives you firm grounds for demanding that your child's academic needs be included in the IEP. Several parents report that one of the best ways to get the rest of your IEP team to understand the problem is using visual aids, such as charts. These can illustrate where your child is at different stages as compared to the norm, or they can compare advances made in the current year to advances made in past years. Sometimes a child who is making very small advances is falling farther and farther behind his peers. If you aren't an artistic whiz, there are software programs that can make simple graphs from your numbers.

Medications at school

Another problem area is the administration of medication at school. Some parents have reported refusal to deliver medication at the appointed time, mysteriously missing pills (especially Ritalin and other amphetamines), and missed or mistaken doses. Most self-contained classrooms have many children who take scheduled medications, and they tend to have processes in place. The worst medication problems seem to occur in full inclusion settings, especially if the student is not capable of monitoring medication delivery himself.

If your child takes medication daily, make sure there is some sort of checklist used to monitor compliance. The person in charge should actually see the child take the medication, not hand it out and let the child walk away. It may be necessary to check the child's mouth to make sure the pills were swallowed. Ask to see the medication compliance checklist at least once a semester, and talk to your child about whether he is getting his meds regularly.

Many children and teens with seizure disorders can take all their meds at home, and this is the best way to avoid school medication problems.

Medications should be properly stored. The pill bottle's label or pharmacy insert should tell you if a medication needs refrigeration or should simply be stored away from light or heat. For safety's sake, medications should be kept in a locked drawer or cabinet. This will protect them from misuse, abuse, and theft. Ask to see where your child's medications will be kept.

If your school has an on-site health clinic or nurse's office, that's probably the best place for your child to get and take his medication. If it does not, someone who is neither licensed nor trained in how to handle medication-related problems will give out medications. This is a dilemma for families whose children need to take medication at school, and for school personnel. School secretaries and teachers are frequently pressed into the role of pill-pushers, and it's rarely one that they relish. Incidentally, in hospitals and nursing homes, a Certified Medication Aide (CMA) license is the minimum qualification required for giving medications to patients.

Schools these days are very concerned about student drug use. School drug policies usually prohibit student possession of prescription and over-the-counter drugs, as well as illicit drugs. Make sure you have a copy of the school's policy on using prescription and non-prescription medications to avoid problems.

It is very rare for even a teenager to be allowed to self-administer medication at school. The usual exceptions to this rule are medications to treat life-threatening symptoms that could emerge suddenly, such as emergency asthma inhalers or an anaphylactic shock kit for students with severe allergies. Medications other than these must usually be kept and administered by a school employee.

Emergency psychiatric medications, including anti-epilepsy medications that can be used on an as-needed basis, are problematic for schools. Unless the school has a medical person on staff, they will naturally be unsure of when to allow your child access to these meds. Ask your physician to write a brief statement about when school personnel should give the medication. Alternatively, you could write this statement yourself. Older children and teens should know the symptoms that these drugs can help with and be able to ask for them independently.

Students may be prescribed medications by a psychiatrist working at the school, with parental permission. Occasionally someone without a license to practice medicine, such as a psychologist or school counselor, may tell pabrents that their child should take a certain medication. In the case of childhood seizure disorders, it's best to have all medication prescribed and managed by someone with considerable expertise in epileptology, a category that few school psychiatrists fall into. Parents do have the right to refuse medication suggested for their child by school personnel, and to ask for a second opinion.

From hospital to school

Imagine how it must feel to be sent to a hospital for a period of a couple weeks or months, then dropped back into your old school as if nothing had happened. You may feel embarrassed. Your medications may make you feel different. If you have had surgery (to implant a vagus nerve stimulation device, for example), your friends may ask embarrassing questions. Everything probably feels very strange.

Nevertheless, every day children and teens are released from the hospital and expected to handle this sudden transition with little support other than encouraging words.

It's best to make the transition from hospital to school a gradual one, starting with a few days or weeks of homebound instruction, then going back to school in a resource room (perhaps with pull-outs for some inclusion activities), half-days at school, or an intermediate period in day treatment. Making a slow transition improves your child's chances for successful reintegration. Think of a best-case scenario and one or more fall-back positions, just in case.

As soon as you begin planning a hospitalization, or when your child enters the hospital if it is a crisis situation, start planning for this transition. Communication is the key. As discussed in the section "Hospital-based education" earlier in this chapter, the school and the hospital must be talking to each other (and to you) from the start. Ask the professionals working with your child in the hospital what they would recommend. They have seen many children your child's age and may have some good ideas.

Identify one person at your child's school—a teacher, counselor, school psychologist, or perhaps an administrator—who can be in charge of the transition back to school. If you have to personally explain the situation to too many people, it's likely that someone will be missed, or that someone will miss out on important information. Preferably this person you choose to be in charge will be someone your child can confide in if problems crop up.

Make sure that both you and your child's school are fully informed about any medications he takes, how they should be administered, and possible side effects. You may also need to adjust the school program to help your child cope with the effects of medication (such as cognitive dulling, sleepiness, or agitation).

Taking on the school system

If your child's school persistently refuses to comply with her IEP, what can you do? A lot—the IEP is a type of legal contract, although far too many schools treat it like a nuisance that they can ignore at their leisure. Your options include:

- Sitting back and letting it happen (obviously not recommended)
- Advocating for your child within the classroom and the IEP process

- Bringing in an expert to help you advocate for your child

- Requesting a due process hearing

- Filing a complaint with your state department of education

- Organizing with other parents to advocate for a group of students with similar problems

- Working with other advocates at a legislative level

- Going to court

While some schools and school districts have a well-deserved reputation for venality, most are simply hamstrung by low budgets and lack of knowledge. These are areas where an informed parent can make a difference. You can provide the teacher and administrators with information about educational possibilities, and you can let them know that their resource problems are something to take up with government funding sources, not a reason for mistreating children.

Remember that, as a full member of the IEP team, you have the power to call an IEP meeting whenever one is needed. This will bring together all of the team members to review the document and to compare its requirements with what your child is receiving.

There are times when you will need to bring in an expert. Special educational advocates and self-styled IEP experts are available all over the country. Some of these people work for disability advocacy organizations or disability law firms. Others are freelance practitioners. Some are parents of children with disabilities who have turned their avocation into a career. You will probably have to pay for expert services, unless they are available through your local Epilepsy Foundation chapter or another parent group. Expert services can include researching programs available in your area, connecting you with appropriate resources, helping you write a better IEP, and advocating for your child at IEP meetings and due process hearings. Appendix A, *Resources*, contains several excellent books that discuss these issues in detail.

Due process

The words due process refer to the procedures that are supposed to be followed when a child is being evaluated for special education or receiving special education services. If you or the school has requested that your child be evaluated for special education services, whether or not he has been approved, you are entitled to due process.

A due process hearing is an internal appeals procedure used by school districts to determine whether or not these procedures have been handled properly. Violations that spark a hearing can include small things, like notifying parents of a meeting over the phone rather in writing; or major issues, like using untrained or incompetent personnel to evaluate children, or deliberately denying needed services to save money.

Obviously, every due process case is unique, and each state also has its own due process system. Regulations that they all have in common are:

- Parents must initiate a due process hearing in writing.

- The hearing must take place in a timely fashion.

- Hearings are presided over by an impartial person who does not work for the district.

- Children have the right to stay in the current placement until after the hearing (this is called the "stay put" rule).

- Parents can attend due process hearings and advocate for their child.

- Parents can hire an educational advocate or lawyer to represent them at the due process hearing.

- If the parents use a lawyer and they win, they are entitled to have their legal fees paid by the district.

Some districts offer arbitration or mediation, which are not as formal as a due process hearing. In an arbitration hearing, both parties agree in advance to comply with the arbitrator's ruling. You can't recover your legal fees in arbitration, and your rights are not spelled out in the law. Be very cautious before agreeing to waive your right to a due process hearing in favor of mediation.

However, you can try mediation without waiving your right to due process while you're waiting for your due process hearing date to come up. If mediation works, you can cancel the due process hearing; if not, you can go ahead with it.

Section 504 actions

You can bypass the cumbersome due process procedure if your child has a 504 plan rather than or in addition to an IEP. Assuming that the school and then the district 504 compliance officer do not respond to your written complaints, take your case directly to your state office of civil rights. This office is responsible for enforcing the Rehabilitation Act.

The state office of civil rights is also charged with enforcing the Americans with Disabilities Act (see the section "Epilepsy and your rights" in Chapter 3).

Public advocacy

If your child is denied special education services, you'll soon find out that you have a lot of company. Some problems in special education are systemic. Parents in several states have banded together effectively to get better services for their children. See Appendix A for a list of support and advocacy groups that may be able to help.

You may choose to form your own organization, join an existing group covering special education issues, or work with a larger group of special education parents. You may also find allies in teachers' unions and organizations, the PTA and other parent associations, and elsewhere in your community.

Parents can personally help improve school funding for special education by lobbying their local school board or state legislature. They can help write and press for laws that require adequate support for these students and for others in the special education system.

If you're not the kind of person who enjoys conflict, advocacy and due process can be very draining. School district lawyers wear down your defenses with endless meetings, criticism of your parenting skills, and constant references to their superior knowledge. You must always stay on guard, and yet be open to logical compromises and the possibility of beneficial alliances. It's not easy, but it's necessary.

Going to court

Going to court is absolutely, positively your last recourse. It's something you do only when nothing else works. It is usually time-consuming, exhausting, and expensive. The outcome is uncertain, and while the case drags on, your child may be languishing in an inappropriate setting. But if you've exhausted every other avenue, it may be the only option left.

Most court cases involving special education target school districts that lost a due process hearing and yet persisted in denying the services mandated for a child. A 1994 case, *W.B. v. Matula*, established the right of parents to sue a school on constitutional grounds. The parent of a grade-schooler who was eventually diagnosed with multiple neurological disabilities took her district to court over violation of her child's due process rights and violation of the Fourteenth Amendment of the Constitution, which entitles all citizens to equal protection under the law. To the consternation of school districts everywhere, she won her case, which included a substantial financial judgment (she used the money to pay her massive legal bills and to get her son an appropriate education).

Since the Matula case, school districts have been put on notice that parents of special-needs children can successfully pursue their rights beyond the due process hearing. Besides the grounds used in the Matula case, parents may be able to ask the courts for redress under state education laws or even contract law. There are few legal precedents as of yet, but the number of successful legal challenges is growing. Court battles are underway in almost every state over unavailable, inadequate, or even harmful special education services.

Education in Canada

The Canadian special education process is very similar to that used in the US. Provincial guidelines are set by the national Ministry of Education and governed by the Education Act. However, most educational decisions are made at the regional, district, or school level.

Special education evaluations are done by a team that may include a school district psychologist, a behavior specialist, a special education teacher, other school or district personnel, and in some cases a parent, although inviting parents to participate is not required by law. The evaluation is used as a basis for an IEP. Almost identical to the American document of the same name, the IEP is usually updated yearly, or more frequently if needed. A formal review is required every three years.

Placement options for Canadian students range from home-based instruction to full inclusion. Partial inclusion is increasingly common, as is supported mainstreaming. Students from rural or poorly served areas may be sent to a residential school, or funding may be provided for room and board to allow the student to attend a day program outside of their home area.

If disputes arise between the school or the district and the parents, there is a School Division Decision Review Process available for adjudicating them. The concept known as due process in the US is usually referred to as fundamental justice in Canada.

Education in the UK

When a child in the UK is judged eligible for special education services, he is said to be statemented. This term refers to an IEP-like document called a Statement of Special Educational Needs (SEN). The SEN is developed at the council level by the Local Educational Authority (LEA) and lists the services that a statemented child needs. Usually the team that creates the SEN includes an educational psychologist, a teacher, and the parents. It may also include the family's health visitor or other medical personnel, such as a psychiatrist or child development specialist. Each child's SEN is reviewed and updated annually. Disability advocates strongly urge parents to get expert help with the statementing process.

Your LEA can limit services according to its budget, even if those services are listed as necessary on your child's SEN. Service availability varies widely between LEAs. Some therapeutic services that would be delivered by schools in the US, such as psychiatric care and therapy, are instead obtained through National Health.

School placements in the UK run the gamut from residential schools to specialist "SEN schools" to full inclusion in mainstream schools. There are more residential options available than in the US system due to the English tradition of public schools. (American readers may be confused by this term: in the UK, privately owned schools are known as public schools, while schools run by the LEAs are called government schools.)

Schools working with statemented students operate under a government code of practice that is analogous to, but much weaker than, IDEA in the US. Parents and disability advocates can insist that LEAs follow this code when devising programs for statemented students and can have access to a formal appeals process.

The UK government has recently taken steps toward improving Early Intervention offerings. Currently, EI services are not mandated by law, although they are available in many areas.

Parents report that homeschooling a child with a disability is particularly hard in some parts of the UK. Regular inspection by an Educational Welfare Officer is required, and some of these bureaucrats are not very knowledgeable about health issues that may affect development and learning. Homeschooling parents should be prepared to provide detailed documentation of what they are teaching and how well their child is progressing.

Education in Australia

In Australia, there is only a thin legal framework for the provision of special education services, but in the urban areas where most Australians live, these services are apparently no harder to obtain than they are in the UK.

In larger cities, early intervention services are readily available for children aged six and under. To obtain an EI evaluation, parents should contact the Specialist Children's Services Team at their local Department of Human Services.

Placement options for older children include residential schools (including placement in residential schools located in the UK, for some students), special schools for children with moderate to severe developmental delay or severe behavior disorders, special classrooms for disabled children within regular schools, and the full range of mainstreaming options. "Mix and match" placements that allow students to be mainstreamed for just part of the day are still rare, however.

Australia has federal special education regulations, but each state's Department of Education, Training, and Employment (DETS) is more important. Each DETS provides information, parent services, assistive technology, augmentative communication, special curricula, and many more services for students with disabilities.

Education in New Zealand

Students who qualify for special education services in New Zealand are called "section nined" (old terminology) or "qualified for the Ongoing Resourcing Scheme" (ORS). ORS qualification is currently reserved for those children whose impairment is judged to be high or very high, with the most resources going to the latter group. As of this writing, special education services for early childhood centers and home-based programs are not funded, although speech therapy and similar services can be obtained through the healthcare system. The Ministry of Education sets qualifying guidelines for early childhood and school-age special education services.

Recent news reports indicate that limited local resources and a move to push for full inclusion under the Special Education 2000 program have eliminated many programs previously available in New Zealand's schools. School placement options include a few special schools, attached special education units within regular schools, and a range of inclusion options in mainstream settings. Some students are in residential settings. Under Special Education 2000, more schools have a resource-room-like arrangement rather than self-contained special education units.

Transitioning to adulthood

Teenagers need to assume ever greater responsibility for managing their own medical care as the years go by. It can be hard for parents to let go, especially if they fear their child may stop taking needed medication or take too many chances with their health. And sometimes the relationship between parent and teenager can get in the way: after all, this is the time when most people question their parents' judgment and seek greater independence.

Teens should be encouraged to start a seizure journal (see Appendix B, *Seizure Diary*) to help them track their own symptoms and communicate with doctors about them. A typical journal would have entries for date, time, and duration of each seizure, as well as space to list sensory, physical, and mental effects of each event. There should also be room in the journal for keeping records of medications taken, timing, and dosage.

One of the most important steps you can take as your teen nears adulthood is allowing her to choose her own medical team. Even though she'll no doubt be choosing from a list of those doctors permitted under your health plan, the fact that it's her own choice will make her feel that she's in charge. And that will make going to the doctor with medical questions or worries more likely during early adulthood, a period when quite a few young people try going without medication or other risky activities. She also needs to start getting herself to medical appointments on occasion, learn how to find out about medication side effects, and understand how to get both emergency and routine healthcare.

Preparation for work and higher education should begin as early as possible. Chapter 3 includes a section on transition planning for teens as they get ready for life beyond high school.

Kids, seizures, and social activities

If your child has partial seizures, it can be a difficult thing to explain to their friends and other parents. Your national epilepsy association probably has educational materials available, and these can go a long way toward ensuring that symptoms are understood, accepted, and taken into account.

Gia says:

> We've found that the school staff copes much better with our pre-schooler's partial complex seizures than do family and friends. Our son has regular weekly seizures with symptoms that include clamped lips, drooling and spitting, staring, flushed or white face, mouth noises, and occasional problems breathing. Our family and friends have a very hard time coping. Only one has offered to baby-sit, and a very close relative recently told me, "This stuff scares me. I just can't baby-sit for you."
>
> It's hard, because my husband and I really never get out by ourselves. Even though we prepare our friends and family about what to expect if one should happen on an outing, it's very difficult for them to witness a seizure and then continue on with the plans of the day. School and home daycare providers are used to seizures and they always make every effort to be accommodating and see to it that James gets a nap break and then is brought up to speed on an activity when he's ready, but family members usually have the hardest time.

Respite care can be essential for parents of disabled children. Your local Epilepsy Foundation chapter or a nearby branch of the Easter Seals should be able to help you identify qualified respite providers if you can't use a family member or friend as a sitter.

These groups may also advise you about special camps and social opportunities for children with epilepsy, as Theresa found out:

> My son went to epilepsy camp last summer. I found out about it in an Epilepsy Foundation monthly newsletter. He had a wonderful time. There were lots of adult counselors and they had many physical activities: a rock

wall to climb, archery, swimming, boating, etc. We even qualified for a
full scholarship offered by a pharmaceutical company, so the week at
camp was free.

Information and education are also the foundation for your child's successful participation in school clubs, summer camps, sports programs, and other social activities. Many national organizations involved in youth activities, including the Boy Scouts and Girl Scouts, have disability specialists available in major metropolitan areas or at the national level. They can help you or youth leaders adapt programs to meet the needs of children with disabilities and come up with ideas for integrating them into the larger group. Theresa describes how beneficial sports have been for her son:

Bryce started having seizures after a brain injury when he was 7. He
was a very good athlete up to that point, and although his skills decreased
after the injury, he kept playing sports. He played soccer, baseball, and
basketball until 8th grade in youth sports programs. In our community,
these were not very competitive and any child who signed up could play.
Most seasons, my husband coached, so we didn't need to worry about
Bryce having a seizure at practice or during games. The times he had
another coach, we would explain about the seizures before the season
started and reassure the coach that one of us would always be there to
take care of things should Bryce have a seizure. I would just go to prac-
tices and read a book. My husband and I both attended all games. Bryce
still had some good skills left—for instance a very strong baseball
swing—and he always felt very accomplished. Not once in all these years
has another child on the team made a negative comment. Sports have
been wonderful for Bryce.

It's not a good idea to encourage kids to hide their disorder. It can foster unnecessary feelings of guilt and shame, emotions that harm a child's self-image and can cause them to withdraw from social situations. Parents need to concentrate on what their child can do, providing any supports needed to let him enjoy the same activities as others his age. That often means helping kids find a way to enjoy social activities despite medication side effects, mobility limits, or other symptoms.

Gia explains:

James has had partial complex seizures since he was an infant. After
a lengthy delay in the diagnosis of his optic glioma, he had surgery, was

placed on anticonvulsants, and eventually needed chemotherapy. He took Dilantin initially, and now he is on Tegretol and Neurontin. Often we weigh the additional sedation and slower processing that comes with higher doses against potentially having additional damage to the brain with uncontrolled seizures. We're just now learning not to let these events ruin our plans or routine. We just bring a wagon wherever we go (some people use regular or special strollers for big kids), and let James sleep it off, and then if we're out somewhere, we just let him see whatever it is he's missed when he's up to it, or do whatever it was that he had planned to do.

Even swimming and contact sports are not necessarily off-limits to kids with epilepsy. Follow your doctor's lead on handling safety issues, such as the need for a helmet, injury-prevention training, or extra supervision.

CHAPTER 5

Medical Interventions

FEAR OF BEING IDENTIFIED as an epileptic is one reason that so many people who have seizures avoid seeking medical care, particularly in countries where being publicly identified as a person with epilepsy could have severe social or legal consequences. For others, however, the reason can be bad experiences with previous treatments and lack of information about what's available now.

If you first sought treatment for epilepsy twenty or thirty years ago, you may have only been offered medications that seemed like more trouble than they're worth. Especially if they are given in large doses, barbiturate drugs like phenobarbital (Solfoton, Luminal) can cause extreme sedation and mental dulling, and older anticonvulsants like phenytoin (Dilantin) can have quite unpleasant side effects. Since the best degree of seizure control was often achieved with a mix of these two drugs or others like them, it was sometimes hard for people to stick with their medication regime. This was doubly true for those not experiencing grand mal seizures, who may have felt less pressured about controlling their symptoms in the first place.

Today, there are many more options for seizure control. That's not to say that the barbiturates and older anticonvulsants are no longer used—quite the contrary. These medications are still very valuable. Many people with epilepsy are able to take them with success and without severe problems. But doctors know more now about when these medications should be tried, how to help patients avoid unwanted side effects, and when some of the newer alternatives may be a better choice.

This chapter covers all of the treatment options, with special attention to balancing medication benefits with the side effects that are unfortunately common with anti-epilepsy drugs. Special sections explain a new device called the vagus nerve stimulator, surgery, and new treatments under development. A medically supervised diet for seizure reduction, the ketogenic diet, is discussed in Chapter 6, *Other Interventions*, as are a variety of complementary approaches that may reduce medication side effects.

Treatment goals

The basic goal of epilepsy treatment is seizure prevention. Dr. Anthony Murro, associate professor of neurology and director of the EEG Laboratory at the Medical College of Georgia, explains how top neurologists gauge treatment options:

> *The goal of epilepsy therapy should be to make a person seizure-free, and this goal should be achieved when the person is young.*
>
> *This is not commonly recognized by physicians, and patients develop low expectations of what can be achieved. For example, a 90 percent reduction in seizure frequency—from ten seizures a month to one seizure a month—might seem like a great achievement. However, even with one seizure a month, the person still cannot drive or work without job restrictions. The person remains dependent on others. Social and personal development is hindered.*
>
> *Real improvement in the quality of life occurs when the person becomes seizure-free. In this case, there are no longer driving or job restrictions, and the person becomes a fully functioning, independent person. The common approach today is that if a person is not made seizure free within one to two years using medications, it is appropriate to consider epilepsy surgery.*

Medication may be recommended to you even though you have only had a few seizures. In some cases, as few as two seizures not caused by a known event (such as a head injury or medication) are sufficient for a doctor to feel that medication is needed, especially for children whose development could be interrupted by uncontrolled seizures and for people with health problems that could be aggravated by seizure activity. If two or more unprovoked seizures have occurred, there is a higher risk that there will be more seizures in the future. Repeated seizures may harm the brain if they are left untreated, although the risk varies greatly depending on the type and length of the seizures.

The most commonly used treatment for epilepsy of any type is medication. Drugs used to control seizures are called anti-epileptic drugs, abbreviated as AEDs. There are several families of drugs that can reduce seizure activity, each of which works in a slightly different way. Some have proven to have more benefit for controlling partial and complex partial seizures than others.

Lifestyle changes, such as stress reduction and removing foods from the diet that seem to trigger seizures, are often recommended to complement medication. These are discussed in Chapter 6. Very few people with epilepsy can eliminate seizures using lifestyle changes alone, but these steps may allow you to reduce the amount of medication you take, thereby limiting your side effects and alleviating medication-related health concerns.

Children and adults who do not respond to medication coupled with lifestyle changes, or who do not achieve sufficient seizure reduction, may want to explore some of the more difficult treatment alternatives. These include the ketogenic diet, the vagus nerve stimulator, and brain surgery.

Taking charge

As you go through life as a person with a partial seizure disorder, it helps to stay in charge of your own treatment plan. Many people have grown up thinking of doctors as all-knowing beings whose advice should be taken without question, but the truth is that doctors do make mistakes sometimes. You can catch these mistakes if you form a partnership with your doctor and know what medications and doses are planned. You may find that doctors help you the most when you take an active role in your own care.

One way to take charge of your care is to educate yourself about treatment options. Reading books like this one is a good start, but online or in-person support groups provide a way to learn from other people's experiences. National organizations like the Epilepsy Foundation also publish excellent materials on treatments, including advance data on drug trials and other new treatment options. Contact information for helpful organizations and support groups is contained in Appendix A, *Resources*.

If you are prescribed a drug, make sure that you fully understand how it works, how it should be used, and what foods, drinks, over-the-counter remedies, prescription drugs, and activities you should avoid while taking it. Monitor your general state of health as well as level of seizure control while taking AEDs, and report any significant changes to your doctor right away. Each AED has certain side effects that are known, but everyone's body chemistry is a little different. You may have no side effects or you may experience a drug-related problem that no one else has ever reported.

Finding a doctor you can trust

Chapter 2, *Diagnosis*, discusses finding a specialist who can handle your ongoing care. While good qualifications and recommendations from other patients are the right criteria for choosing a neurologist, epileptologist, or psychiatrist as your primary epilepsy care provider, building an ongoing relationship with that person is the key to quality care.

Ron talks about how important your practitioner is:

> In evaluating treatments, I have one big item—find a doctor who will listen to you! Also, a doctor needs to be able to talk to patients at their level. We aren't medical school graduates, and we don't know all the fancy fourteen-letter words. My current doctor is very good at listening to his patients, and does not throw a lot of fancy terminology at them (unless he defines it first).

Working with your doctor should be a long-term partnership when you have a chronic health condition. One of your top priorities as you embark on a relationship with a new doctor is to make your treatment goals clear. Your doctor needs to know how your seizures affect your daily life, and what you would consider a good quality of life. She needs to know what kinds of medication side effects are acceptable to you given the severity of your seizures, and what side effects are not acceptable. Then you and your doctor can work together toward mutual goals based on these factors.

As treatment continues, evaluate your progress against these goals. Ask your doctor what might be done differently if you are still experiencing too many breakthrough episodes or if side effects are intolerable. Many times people are afraid to bring "minor" medication-related concerns, such as sexual dysfunction or stomachaches, to their doctor's attention. Their dissatisfaction can build until it boils over. You may have to remind yourself occasionally that when it comes to quality of life issues, nothing is too minor to mention. The solution may be as simple as a change in medication or even just taking your medication with food.

Jim discusses how doctors and patients may not see eye-to-eye about side effects:

> Out of all the problems and challenges I have experienced, the most troublesome for me are those related to cognitive disruptions and challenges. It is frequently remarked in the literature on seizures that most such challenges make a "negligible" difference in the life of the patient. Such remarks are usually made concerning the results of neurological testing and the statistics derived from these tests, alone or combined with other information and/or testing results. Well, actually living with "negligible" differences of cognition may not seem like a minor thing for the person being forced to live with the difference.

> For example, a 5 percent reduction in cognitive ability may be considered a negligible difference, but I have little doubt that the professionals saying and believing this would be in a real panic if all of a sudden they were to experience a very real 5 percent decrease in their cognitive functions. For many professionals, this would mean an abrupt end to their career.

Complete seizure control is not always possible. The amount of medication needed for optimal seizure control often causes other problems that are just as debilitating as the seizures themselves. Always keeping the goal of neuroprotection in mind, work with your doctor to find a balance between seizure effects and medication effects.

How seizure medications work

The drugs prescribed to control seizures come from several different families of chemicals. All of them are active inside the brain, but surprisingly not much is known about how they actually work. Current theories hold that AEDs may help in the following ways:

- Limiting the repeated firing of electrical charges by neurons, as sodium (Na+) channel blockers can do
- Enhancing the effects of the neurotransmitter gamma-aminobutyric acid (GABA), which also limits neuronal firing
- Reducing the activity level of voltage-sensitive calcium (Ca++) channels, as calcium channel blockers do
- Decreasing the general level of neuronal excitement in the brain, a process mediated by chemicals called glutamates

Blocking the Na+ channel limits neurotransmitter production, including the neurotransmitters that may be involved in increases in neuronal firing. It seems to stabilize the membranes of neurons, calming down electrical and chemical activity. AEDs known to inhibit the Na+ channel include Dilantin, Tegretol, Lamictal, Trileptal, Topamax, Neurontin, Felbatol, Depakote, and Depakene.

Blocking one type of calcium channel seems to be very effective in treating absence seizures, while blocking another high-voltage calcium channel appears more effective for preventing partial seizures. When calcium channels are blocked, neurotransmitter release is reduced. High levels of calcium within brain cells are also believed to trigger a series of processes that can lead to cell death and brain damage, so medications that block calcium channels may have extra neuroprotective effects. This group includes Zarontin, Depakote, Depakene, Zonegran, Felbatol, Lamictal, Topamax, and Neurontin.

Only a few AEDs affect glutamate receptors in the brain. Phenobarbital inhibits one type of glutamate receptor (though that's not its primary method of antiseizure activity), while Felbatol and Topamax affect another. Phenobarbital and other barbiturate tranquilizers are also muscle relaxants, although this does not have an impact on seizures.

Quite a few medications appear to affect the activity of GABA in the brain, particularly the benzodiazepine tranquilizers, such as Valium. Some AEDs are thought to mimic GABA's inhibitory action or increase the amount of GABA that's active in the brain, including phenobarbital, Neurontin, Felbatol, Gabitril, Sabril, Zonegran, and possibly Depakote and Depakene.[1]

Anti-epilepsy drugs (AEDs)

This section lists and briefly describes all of the most commonly used AEDs, in alphabetical order according to their best-known US brand name. Most people with seizure disorders can find adequate relief from a single medication (monotherapy), and this is the goal doctors usually work toward when prescribing. Others respond better to a combination of two or more medications, carefully balanced to address individual symptoms without causing unbearable side effects.

If you do take more than one medication, even if they are for different health problems, pay very close attention to information on how drugs can affect each other. Anti-anxiety drugs and sleeping pills pose a particular risk when taken with AEDs, as do some other types of drugs. For example, Valium combined with Depakote can be quite dangerous, and some blood-pressure medications are counteracted by phenobarbital.

Over-the-counter drugs can also pose interaction hazards. As you look over the list of AEDs in this chapter, you'll notice that some should not be mixed with aspirin, antacids like Alka-Seltzer, and medications that contain stimulants, such as many non-prescription allergy remedies. Most people who take AEDs also need to avoid alcohol. Be sure to talk to your doctor about this and other restrictions.

Before taking a new medication, discuss it thoroughly with your doctor, and read the package insert that comes with it. You may also want to consult a medicine reference book, several of which are listed in Appendix A. Only the most common side effects and cautions are listed here. You may experience rare side effects, or even problems that no other patient has reported. If you experience unusual symptoms after taking medicine, or after combining more than one medication, call your doctor right away.

Jacky, age 39, has temporal lobe epilepsy. She is all too familiar with medication side effects and hazards:

> I am on Tegretol and Neurontin, and my most troubling side effects
> are double vision, dizziness, and not being able to finish a thought with-
> out forgetting what I was about to say! I have poor short-term memory,
> although that may be due to the seizures. Side effects are probably the
> main reason people fail to comply with their medical regime. I get real
> bad days when I think it just can't be worth it, but then I think how much
> worse off I'd be if I were actively seizing all the time.

Many medications are available in less-expensive generic forms, while others are not (although all have a generic chemical name). Generics are supposed to be identical to the brand name drugs they are based on, but doctors have found that some generic AEDs are significantly different. For that reason, if you switch from a brand name to a generic, pay close attention just as you would when taking a totally new drug. Also, watch out for changes in the generic itself—many different companies can make generic medications, and while Company A's version may work well for you, Company B's may not.

Most of the medications listed in this chapter are available in the US and Canada. Brand names and formulations may vary in other countries, and some drugs may not be available elsewhere.

Sometimes medications that have not been formally approved by government regulators are available under "compassionate use" laws designed to make sure needy patients do not go without access to promising medications, including drugs that normally would only be available overseas. Ask your physician about how to apply for compassionate use approval. Sometimes a physician in one country can prescribe a medication available only overseas, and patients can then have the prescription filled at an overseas pharmacy. Investigate the regulations prior to trying to import medications.

A number of promising new AEDs are under development, and some of these as-yet-unapproved drugs are sometimes given to participants in human research trials. If you don't have success with any of the usual treatments for your seizures, do consider pursuing this avenue.

The US National Institutes of Health (NIH) runs many clinical trials each year, as do similar health agencies in other countries, university-linked research centers, and some pharmaceutical companies. Your nearest major research hospital is a good place to learn more about drug trials in your area, as are the Epilepsy Foundation and local epilepsy support groups. Clinical trials are also listed on the NIH site (*http://clinicaltrials.gov/ct/gui/*) and at CenterWatch (*http://www.centerwatch.com*). See Appendix A for more information on clinical trials.

The information in this chapter is taken from the *Physician's Desk Reference*, pharmaceutical company literature, and other reputable sources. It is accurate as of this writing, but new information may emerge. Because AEDs do have a high potential for side effects and interactions with other medications, it's important to know as much as possible about drugs you are prescribed or that you may hear about. A drug that has gotten bad reviews from others may turn out to be perfect for you. Similarly, what works well for someone in your support group may not work well for you.

Pat says the medication side effects she has experienced made her look more closely at medication alternatives:

> When I was first diagnosed with epilepsy at age 21, the doctor I was seeing prescribed Dilantin and phenobarbital. I had a hard time concentrating, fatigued easily, and felt very groggy in the mornings. Sometimes,

for no apparent reason, a glass would slip out of my hands. I think this was due to the pheno, because the next neurologist I went to took me off pheno and I felt much better.

Anti-epilepsy drug list

Drugs used to treat partial complex seizures are known by a variety of names. You may hear the same drug referred to by its generic name, abbreviation, or one of several brand names. The following table gives the most common names used for antiseizure drugs and tells you what name is used in this chapter so you can easily find it on the following pages of detailed information:

Name	Look Under
Apo-catazolimide	Diamox
Apo-carbamazepine	Tegretol
Carbamazepine	Tegretol
Cerebyx	Cerebyx
Clonazepam	Klonopin
Convulex	Depakote
Depakene	Depakene
Depakote	Depakote
Diamox	Diamox
Dilantin	Dilantin
Divalproex sodium	Depakote
Epilim	Depakote
Epitol	Tegretol
Ethotoin	Peganone
Ethosuximide	Zarontin
Excegran	Zonegran
Felbamate	Felbatol
Felbatol	Felbatol
Fosphenytoin	Cerebyx
Gabapentin	Neurontin
Gabitril	Gabitril
Keppra	Keppra
Klonopin	Klonopin
Lamictal	Lamictal
Lamotrigine	Lamictal
Levetiracetam	Keppra
Mogadon	Nitrazadon

Name	Look Under
Neurontin	Neurontin
Nitrazadon	Nitrazadon
Oxcarbazepine	Trileptal
Peganone	Peganone
Phenobarbital	Phenobarbital
Phenytoin	Dilantin
Rivotril	Klonopin
Sabril	Sabril
Tegretol	Tegretol
Topamax	Topamax
Topiramate	Topamax
Tiagabine hydrochloride	Gabitril
Trileptal	Trileptal
Valproate	Depakote
Valproic acid	Depakene
Vigabatrin	Sabril
Zarontin	Zarontin
Zonegran	Zonegran
Zonisamide	Zonegran

Cerebyx

Generic name: Fosphenytoin

Use: Seizure disorders, especially local-focal (grand mal) seizures. Cerebyx is given intravenously as an emergency treatment for seizures—it is not a medication that is used on a regular basis or outside of a hospital setting.

Action, if known: Cerebyx is a hydantoin AED, which inhibits activity in the part of the brain where local-focal seizures begin.

Side effects: Common side effects of Cerebyx include gum growth, confusion, twitching, depression, and irritability.

Known interaction hazards: The effects of Cerebyx are increased by alcohol, aspirin, sulfa drugs, succinimide antiseizure medications, some neuroleptics and antidepressants, and many other drugs. Cerebyx increases the effects of lithium, acetaminophen, and many other drugs. Using calcium supplements, antacids, charcoal tablets, and many prescription drugs will change the effectiveness of Cerebyx. If you have grand mal seizures that could lead to emergency treatment, be sure to wear a medical alert bracelet or carry a wallet card that lists the medications you use, so that emergency care personnel can adjust the dose of Cerebyx or other medications they use accordingly.

Tips: Cerebyx is not recommended for use by people who have low blood pressure or heart trouble. Contact your doctor if you develop a skin rash or bruising after treatment with Cerebyx, as these can be serious warning signs.

Depakene

Generic name: Valproic acid

Use: Seizure disorders, bipolar disorders, migraine, panic disorder, rages/aggression.

Action, if known: Depakene increases the level and absorption of GABA in the brain. It stabilizes brain membranes, preventing activity that may contribute to seizures.

Side effects: Common side effects of Depakene are nausea, sedation, depression, psychosis, aggression, hyperactivity, and changes in blood platelet function.

Known interaction hazards: Do not take Depakene with milk, and avoid taking charcoal tablets when taking this drug. Alcohol or any medication that has a tranquilizing or depressant effect should be avoided. Side effects may increase if you use anticoagulants, including aspirin; non-steroidal anti-inflammatory drugs; erythromycin; Thorazine and similar neuroleptics; Tagamet (cimetidine) and other histamine blockers; or Felbatol.

Tips: Watch out for increased bruising or bleeding, an indicator of blood platelet problems. Do not crush or chew tablets. Starting with a very small dose and titrating it up slowly can often help patients avoid even the common side effects. When pregnant women take this medication, their offspring run a higher risk of the birth defect spina bifida. If you are pregnant or could become pregnant, talk to your doctor about taking folic acid supplements and/or changing your treatment plan temporarily to reduce this risk. (See also the tips for Depakote, all of which also apply to Depakene.)

Depakote, Depakote Sprinkles

Generic name: Divalproex sodium (valproic acid plus sodium valproate). Convulex is a brand name available in Europe, UK, and South Africa. Epilim is a brand name available in UK, Australia, and New Zealand.

Use: Seizure disorders, bipolar disorders, migraine, panic disorder, rages/ aggression.

Action, if known: Depakote increases the level of GABA in the brain, and increases its absorption. It stabilizes brain membranes.

Side effects: Side effects include nausea, sedation (this usually passes after a few days), depression, psychosis, aggression, hyperactivity, changes in blood platelet function, hair loss. Depakote causes a 1 to 2 percent risk of spina bifida in children born to mothers who take this drug.

Known interaction hazards: Both milk and charcoal tablets can interfere with the action of this drug. Alcohol or any medication that has a tranquilizing or depressant effect should be avoided. Side effects may increase if you use anticoagulants, including aspirin; non-steroidal anti-inflammatory drugs; erythromycin; Thorazine (chlorpromazine) and similar neuroleptics; Tagamet (cimetidine); or Felbatol.

Tips: Watch out for increased bruising or bleeding, an indicator of blood platelet problems. Regular liver tests are sometimes recommended while taking this drug, particularly for patients who are younger than two years of age. Depakote has recently been linked to polycystic ovaries in female patients. The symptoms of this problem include irregular periods and unexplained weight gain. Do not crush or chew tablets. Starting with a very small dose and slowly increasing it over time can often help patients avoid even the common side effects—the Depakote Sprinkles version is often a good choice for doing this. Hair loss due to Depakote may be avoided by taking 50 mg of zinc daily; some patients also take .025 mg of selenium to boost zinc's effect. Depakote may also interfere with how the body processes carnitine, a protein that can affect energy level, metabolism, and weight. Carnitine levels can be tested, and a prescription supplement (Carnitor) is available. When pregnant women take this medication, there is a higher risk of the birth defect spina bifida in their infants. If you are pregnant or could become pregnant, talk to your doctor about taking folic acid supplements and/or changing your treatment plan temporarily to reduce this risk.

Diamox

Generic name: Acetazolamide

Use: Seizure disorders, particularly absence seizures.

Action, if known: Diamox inhibits the enzyme carbonic anhydrase.

Side effects: Side effects include nausea, tingling, decreased appetite and weight, increased urination, drowsiness, and increased sensitivity to sunlight may occur when taking Diamox.

Known interaction hazards: Prescription or over-the-counter stimulants, cyclosporine, Mysoline, and aspirin may interact with Diamox.

Tips: Do not take Diamox if you are allergic to sulfa drugs. This drug is less likely to upset your stomach if taken with food. It tends to cause potassium loss, so supplementation is sometimes necessary.

Dilantin

Generic name: Phenytoin

Use: Seizure disorders, particularly tonic-clonic seizures.

Action, if known: Dilantin is a hydantoin AED, and it inhibits activity in the part of the brain where tonic-clonic seizures begin.

Side effects: Side effects include gum growth, confusion, twitching, depression, irritability, excessive hair growth, and many more side effects have been associated with Dilantin, some of which are very serious. Due to the many interaction problems with this drug, discuss it thoroughly with your doctor and pharmacist before use.

Known interaction hazards: Dilantin's effects may be increased by alcohol, aspirin, sulfa drugs, succinimide antiseizure medications, some neuroleptics and antidepressants, and many other drugs. It increases the effects of lithium, Tylenol (acetaminophen), and many other drugs. Its effects are changed by use of calcium, antacids, charcoal tablets, and many prescription drugs. Dilantin can cause irregular bleeding when taken with oral contraceptives, and it can also cause oral contraceptive failure, leading to unplanned pregnancy. Switching to an oral contraceptive with greater estrogen content may prevent this problem.

Tips: Contact your doctor if you develop a skin rash or bruising, which can be serious warning signs. You may want to supplement with folic acid, which is depleted by Dilantin. Regular blood tests are recommended while taking this drug to reduce the risk of heart problems. Take with food if stomach upset occurs—but not with high-calcium foods, such as dairy products, sesame seeds, or some nuts. The distressing gum problems associated with Dilantin (and sometimes with other AEDs) can often be avoided with a special program of dental care, including flossing, regular professional cleaning, and possibly a special mouthwash that includes folic acid—ask your dentist for advice. Do not switch brands of generic phenytoin without telling your doctor.

Felbatol

Generic name: Felbamate

Use: Seizure disorders.

Action, if known: Felbatol raises the seizure threshold. It also relaxes the muscles, although this does not have an impact on seizure activity.

Side effects: Felbatol can cause insomnia, fatigue, tremor, anxiety, headache, or increased sun sensitivity. Aplastic anemia, a potentially life-threatening reduction in white and red blood cells, is also associated with Felbatol.

Known interaction hazards: Felbatol breaks down Tegretol, but it prevents Dilantin from breaking down.

Tips: Felbatol is considered one of the more dangerous AEDs and should only be tried when others have failed. Regular blood tests are recommended during the first year, when those susceptible to aplastic anemia are most likely to develop it. One advantage to Felbatol is that it normally doesn't affect lithium levels, so it may be an appropriate choice for a person with both bipolar disorder and partial seizures who has been stabilized on lithium.

Gabitril

Generic name: Tiagabine hydrochloride (HCL)

Use: Seizure disorders, including partial seizure disorders.

Action, if known: Gabitril enhances the activity of GABA and may have other as yet unknown effects.

Side effects: This medication can cause dizziness, drowsiness, nausea, irritability, tremor, stomach problems, severe rash, weakness, and uncontrolled eye movements. It can lower your white blood cell and blood platelet count.

Known interaction hazards: Antacids should not be taken with Gabitril, and hepatic enzyme-inducing AEDs like Tegretol may counteract it. Gabitril may interact with other AEDs as well, so always monitor dosage carefully to avoid toxic reactions.

Tips: Gabitril is used mostly in addition to other AEDs. It is not yet recommended for use by children under 12.

Keppra

Generic name: Levetiracetam

Use: Simple and complex partial seizures; may also be effective for myoclonic and other types of seizures.

Action, if known: Keppra is believed to bind to a specific site in the plasma membranes of brain synapses, inhibiting burst firing by neurons but not normal firing.

Side effects: Side effects include drowsiness, fatigue, impaired coordination, and unusual behavior may occur when taking Keppra.

Known interaction hazards: No important interaction hazards have been identified as of yet.

Tips: Keppra is currently recommended for use only in addition to other AEDs. People with kidney problems should be monitored closely when using Keppra and may want to avoid this medication. Keppra was just approved for use by adults in the US as this book went to press, and it had not yet been approved in Canada. It has been available in some parts of Europe for a few years, however. Early reports indicate that patients can start on a therapeutic dose of Keppra without harm, rather than moving up slowly from a lower one.

Klonopin

Generic name: Clonazepam. Rivotril is a brand name available in Europe and Asia.

Use: Seizure disorders, panic attacks, restless leg syndrome, acute mania and manic psychosis, schizophrenia, chronic pain, speech problems from Parkinson's disease.

Action, if known: Klonopin depresses the central nervous system in order to raise the seizure threshold. It also relaxes muscles, although this does not have an impact on seizure activity.

Side effects: Klonopin can cause drowsiness, unusual behavior, and difficulty controlling muscles. This medication is addictive, and withdrawal may be difficult.

Known interaction hazards: Klonopin may interact with Depakene or Depakote. This drug may also interact with other AEDs, so use it alone or make sure your use of AEDs is carefully monitored. Avoid alcohol, narcotics, tranquilizers, CNS depressants, MAOI antidepressants, and tricyclic antidepressants. Do not take Klonopin with antacids. Klonopin can increase the effects of digoxin. Its own effect is increased by the antihistamine Tagamet (cimetidine), the antifungal drug Nizoral (ketoconazole), probenecid (found in the antibiotic Probampacin, among other places), the painkiller Darvon (propoxyphene), the beta-blockers Inderal (propranolol) and Lopressor/Toprol (metoprolol), and the antibiotic rifampin, as well as similar drugs. Klonopin works against the effects of L-dopa.

Tips: You will need regular blood and liver function tests while taking Klonopin. Smoking or using the nicotine patch may interfere with its effectiveness. People tend to build up a tolerance to this drug quickly, so your dose may need to be changed frequently.

Lamictal

Generic name: Lamotrigine

Use: Seizure disorders, including simple and complex partial seizures; Lennox-Gastaut syndrome in children; bipolar disorders.

Action, if known: Lamictal binds to the hormone melatonin. It stabilizes electrical currents within the brain and blocks the release of seizure-stimulating neurotransmitters. Lamictal is believed to have greater neuroprotective abilities than some other AEDs.[2]

Side effects: Lamictal can cause headache, dizziness, nausea, a general flu-like feeling, and increased light sensitivity. If you develop a rash, call your doctor immediately, as it may be a warning of a serious, even life-threatening, side effect. The likelihood of this problem is especially high in children. Lamictal may make seizures worse in some people.

Known interaction hazards: Lamictal interacts with Depakote/Depakene, Tegretol, and Dilantin—your doctor will have to monitor doses carefully. Antifolate drugs increase its action. Solfoton and Mysoline may lessen its effects. Lamictal can cause irregular bleeding when taken with oral contraceptives, and it can also cause oral contraceptive failure, leading to unplanned pregnancy. Switching to an oral contraceptive with greater estrogen content may prevent this problem.

Tips: Lamictal is not normally recommended for use by children, except in cases of Lennox-Gastaut syndrome, although some neurologists have found it useful for other forms of pediatric epilepsy. If you have heart, kidney, or liver disease, use this drug only under careful supervision. Lamictal sometimes has an antidepressant effect when used with another AED or lithium. It is usually used in addition to other medication rather than as monotherapy.

Neurontin

Generic name: Gabapentin

Use: Seizure disorders, especially those that do not respond to other drugs; anxiety; panic; bipolar disorders; rage/aggression.

Action, if known: This AED appears to act by binding to a specific protein found only on neurons in the central nervous system. It may increase the GABA content of some brain regions.

Side effects: Side effects include blurred vision, dizziness, clumsiness, drowsiness, swaying, and eye-rolling have been associated with Neurontin. It can also cause edema (swelling caused by water retention) in the legs.

Known interaction hazards: Avoid alcohol and all other central nervous system depressants, including tranquilizers, over-the-counter medications for colds and allergies, sleep aids, anesthetics, and narcotics while taking this drug. Antacids may counteract the effects of Neurontin.

Tips: Start with a very low dose and raise slowly to avoid side effects. People with kidney disease should be carefully monitored while taking Neurontin. Corn is used as a filler in the usual formulation of this drug, causing allergic reactions in some. Recent reports indicate that Neurontin can cause mania in some patients, especially children. This can be offset by adding another medication, or by changing the dose of Neurontin or other medications used with it. Others report that Neurontin made their psoriasis worse. A new drug under development called Pregabolin is based on Neurontin, but with fewer side effects.

Nitrazadon

Generic name: Nitrazepam. This drug is available in Canada, the UK, Australia, New Zealand, Asia, and Europe, but not the US.

Use: Myoclonic seizures, infantile spasms.

Action, if known: A benzodiazepine tranquilizer, Nitrazadon depresses CNS activity to raise the seizure threshold. It also relaxes muscles, although this does not have an impact on seizure activity.

Side effects: Side effects include fatigue, sleepiness, loss of coordination, and mental confusion have been associated with Nitrazadon.

Known interaction hazards: Avoid alcohol and any other CNS depressant while taking Nitrazadon, which may also interact with some other AEDs.

Tips: People with kidney or liver problems should be closely monitored when taking Nitrazadon. You may have headaches for a while after you stop taking this drug. Nitrazadon is often given in combination with steroids.

Peganone

Generic name: Ethotoin

Use: Seizure disorders.

Action, if known: Peganone, a hydantoin AED, inhibits activity in the part of the brain where local-focal seizures begin.

Side effects: Side effects include gum growth, confusion, twitching, depression, irritability, and many more side effects may occur when taking Peganone, some of which are very serious. Due to the many interaction problems with this drug, discuss it thoroughly with your doctor and pharmacist.

Known interaction hazards: The effect of Peganone is increased by alcohol, aspirin, sulfa drugs, succinimide antiseizure medications, some neuroleptics and antidepressants, and many other drugs. It strengthens the effect of lithium, acetaminophen, and many other drugs. Its effects are changed by use of calcium, antacids, charcoal tablets, and many prescription drugs.

Tips: Peganone is not usually recommended for people who have low blood pressure or heart trouble. Keep an eye out for skin rash or bruising, which can be serious warning signs. You may want to supplement with folic acid, which is depleted by Peganone. You may need to have regular blood tests while taking this drug. Take your medicine with food if stomach upset occurs—but not with high-calcium foods, such as dairy products, sesame seeds, or some nuts. Do not switch brands without telling your doctor.

Phenobarbital

Generic name: Phenobarbital

Use: Seizure disorder, insomnia.

Action, if known: As a barbiturate, phenobarbital blocks or slows nerve impulses in the brain. It is usually used in combination with another drug to control seizures.

Side effects: High doses of phenobarbital can produce an effect that looks (and feels) like alcohol or drug intoxication. You may experience drowsiness, slow reflexes, and labored breathing. Call your doctor if any side effect becomes bothersome, or if you develop anemia or jaundice. This drug carries an addiction risk, so taper off your dose carefully under medical supervision if stopping its use.

Known interaction hazards: Alcohol, MAOIs, and Depakote or Depakene all increase the effect of phenobarbital. This drug is neutralized by charcoal, chloramphenicol, and rifampin. It increases the effect of Tylenol (acetaminophen) and the anesthetic methoxyflurane, and changes how many other drugs act in the body, including anticoagulants, beta-blockers, and corticosteroids. Phenobarbital can cause irregular bleeding when taken with oral contraceptives, and it can also cause oral contraceptive failure, leading to unplanned pregnancy. Switching to an oral contraceptive with greater estrogen content may prevent this problem. Be sure to go over all medicines you take with your doctor, as doses may need to be adjusted.

Tips: You may want to supplement with vitamin D when taking phenobarbital. People with liver or kidney disease should be closely monitored when taking this drug.

Sabril

Generic name: Vigabatrin. It is available in Europe and Canada, but not in the US.

Use: Simple and complex partial seizures, Lennox-Gastaut syndrome, infantile spasms.

Action, if known: Sabril increases GABA levels in the brain.

Side effects: Sabril can cause drowsiness, fatigue, nausea, headache, and weight gain. It can also cause vision impairment (including tunnel vision), which may be irreversible. It can cause manic or psychotic episodes in some people (particularly those who have had these episodes before).

Known interaction hazards: Do not use alcohol when taking Sabril. This drug counteracts Dilantin.

Tips: People with kidney problems must be carefully monitored while taking Sabril, and it is not recommended for use by people who have had manic or psychotic episodes. Interestingly, Sabril has also shown promise as a remedy for cocaine addiction. Sabril is normally used in addition to other medications.

Tegretol

Generic name: Carbamazepine. Epitol is a brand name available in Canada.

Use: Seizure disorders (including simple and complex partial seizures), nerve pain, bipolar disorders, rage/aggression, aid to drug withdrawal, restless leg syndrome, Sydenham's chorea and similar disorders in children.

Action, if known: Tegretol appears to work by reducing electrical responses among many synapses in the brain, and has other as yet unknown effects.

Side effects: Tegretol can cause sleepiness, dizziness, nausea, unusual moods or behavior, headache, and retention of water. It may cause low white blood cell count. Call your doctor right away if you have flu-like symptoms or other unusual reactions while taking this drug.

Known interaction hazards: Never take Tegretol with an MAOI antidepressant. Tegretol is often used in combination with other AEDs or lithium, but the doses of Tegretol and any drugs used with it must be very carefully adjusted. The effect of Tegretol is strengthened by numerous prescription and over-the-counter medications, including many antibiotics, antidepressants, and cimetidine. It also counteracts or changes the effect of many drugs, including Haldol, bronchodilators containing theophylline, and Tylenol (acetaminophen). Because these interactions can be very serious, discuss all medications you take—including all non-prescription remedies—with your doctor before beginning to use Tegretol. Tegretol can cause irregular bleeding when taken with oral contraceptives, and it can also cause oral contraceptive failure, leading to unplanned pregnancy. Switching to an oral contraceptive with greater estrogen content may prevent this problem.

Tips: You should have a white blood cell count done before taking Tegretol, and some doctors want patients to have this test done occasionally thereafter. A slight reduction in the number of white blood cells is common when using this drug and is not a cause for alarm. This drug probably won't be prescribed if you have a history of bone marrow depression, however. Tegretol can cause serious side effects, so all patients taking this drug should be carefully monitored, particularly since it interacts with so many other medications. In 1998 a warning was issued that liquid Tegretol suspension should not be taken with other liquid or syrup medications due to a potentially dangerous side effect, in which the medications may combine to form a rubbery mass in the bowel.

Topamax

Generic name: Topiramate

Use: Seizure disorders, including as an adjunctive therapy for partial seizure disorders.

Action, if known: Topamax enhances the activity of GABA, acts as a calcium-channel blocker, and blocks the excitatory neurotransmitter glutamate. It may have other, as yet unknown, effects. Topamax is believed to have greater neuroprotective abilities than some other AEDs.[3]

Side effects: Topamax may cause sleepiness, dizziness, loss of coordination, slowed thinking and speech, tingling in the extremities, nausea, tremor, depression, visual disturbances, or increased aggression. Significant mood changes such as irritability and anger occur rather often with this drug.

Known interaction hazards: Alcohol should be avoided when taking Topamax. Adjust dosages carefully when using this drug with other AEDs or any CNS depressant drug. Topamax reduces the effectiveness of digoxin. It can cause irregular bleeding when taken with oral contraceptives and may also cause oral contraceptive failure, leading to unplanned pregnancy. Switching to an oral contraceptive with greater estrogen content may prevent this problem.

Tips: Topamax was recently approved for use in children as young as age two who have partial seizures, and it is available in a "sprinkle" formulation that can be combined with soft food, such as applesauce. Because of the side effects that can happen with this drug, it is recommended that people start with very low doses and increase the dose upward very slowly. People with kidney or liver problems should be closely monitored while taking Topamax.

Trileptal

Generic name: Oxcarbazepine

Use: Partial seizure disorders, both as monotherapy for adults and as a secondary medication for adults or children.

Action, if known: Trileptal is believed to work by blockading voltage-sensitive sodium channels in the brain.

Side effects: Trileptal can cause dizziness, drowsiness, fatigue, nausea, headache, or vision impairment.

Known interaction hazards: Alcohol, other CNS depressants, and calcium-channel blockers like Plendil interact with Trileptal. This drug counteracts birth control pills.

Tips: Another very recently approved AED, Trileptal can be used in patients as young as 4. It is somewhat similar chemically to Tegretol, so if you have problems with that AED, Trileptal may not be a good choice. It can cause low sodium levels in some patients.

Zarontin

Generic name: Ethosuximide

Use: Absence (petit mal) seizure disorders.

Action, if known: Zarontin is a succinimide AED.

Side effects: Side effects include nausea, abdominal cramps, changes in appetite, weight loss, drowsiness, headache, dizziness, irritability, and insomnia may occur when taking Zarontin. This medication may lower the seizure threshold in some patients with mixed forms of epilepsy.

Known interaction hazards: Zarontin increases the effects of Cerebyx, Dilantin, and Peganone.

Tips: You should have regular liver function and blood tests while taking this drug. Zarontin may cause systemic lupus erythematosus (a medication-caused form of the auto-immune disorder lupus).

Zonegran

Generic name: Zonisamide

Use: Partial seizure disorders and seizures that occur during sleep. Zonegran is currently recommended for use with other AEDs.

Action, if known: Zonegran is believed to block sodium channels in the brain, stabilizing neuronal membranes. This may prevent inflammation as well as block seizure activity. It does not seem to affect GABA, but it does increase the amount of active serotonin and dopamine in the brain.

Side effects: Side effects include tiredness, nausea, headache, irritability, agitated behavior, poor concentration, and weight loss may occur when taking Zonegran.

Known interaction hazards: Zonegran does not seem to affect plasma levels of other AEDs, but its effectiveness may be decreased by Solfoton, Dilantin, or Tegretol.

Tips: Do not take Zonegran if you are allergic to sulfa drugs. People with kidney or liver problems should be carefully monitored. Zonegran is one of the newest AEDs for use in the US and Europe, although it has been available in Japan since 1989.

Other medications

There are two major types of medications that may be added to an AED to treat partial complex seizures: benzodiazepine tranquilizers used on an as-needed basis (or in some cases regularly) and steroids. Using either of these is not a decision to take lightly. Both have a high potential for side effects, even more so than some of the AEDs. However, for certain types of seizures and for certain patients, adding these drugs can greatly improve seizure control and quality of life.

Benzodiazepine tranquilizers

Drugs in the benzodiazepine family are sometimes called minor tranquilizers (as compared to barbiturates like phenobarbital, the major tranquilizers), although there's nothing minor about the way they make you feel—slow, tired, and foggy. Normally prescribed for patients with severe anxiety, these medications also have a place in epilepsy treatment because they increase the brain-calming action of GABA. Other than the benzodiazepines listed in the previous section on AEDs, drugs in this family are most frequently used for emergency room treatment of status epilepticus. They may also be prescribed on an as-needed basis to patients whose seizures get worse in times of severe anxiety and stress, or who simply have breakthrough seizures on occasion.

All of the benzodiazepines can be addictive. They all also have a high potential for interacting with AEDs, so your doctor will need to choose doses carefully. They should never be used in conjunction with alcohol or any other depressant drug—death can result from such combinations.

Side effects with any of these medicines include drowsiness, confusion, loss of muscle coordination, weakness, slurred speech, memory problems, and urine retention. People with kidney or liver problems must be carefully monitored when taking these medications, and blood tests are necessary for long-term users.

Iain has experienced some of the more difficult side effects associated with AEDs:

> *Phenytoin did awful things to my gums. It exposed the nerves at the bottom and top of the teeth and gave me a lot of pain.*

> *At one point my Tegretol dose went up too high in an effort to kill the seizures and I got double vision, a splitting headache, and became very unstable on my feet. I basically took matters into my own hands. I cut the dose back and made another appointment ASAP.*

The following are some of the most frequently used benzodiazepines:

- Ativan (lorazepam).

- Frisium (clobazam). Not yet approved in the US, Frisium is prescribed in Canada as a maintenance drug for seizure disorders, including partial seizures. It is almost always used in addition to another AED. Taking Frisium with food should minimize any nausea.

- Librium (chlordiazepoxide, also known as Tropium).

- Valium (diazepam, also known as Atensine, Diazemuls, Rimaprim, Tensium, Vivol). Valium can be administered as a pill, liquid, injectable, or rectal gel (Diastat), and it is probably the most common medication used for emergency hospital treatment of people with epilepsy. Diastat gel may be used at home under some circumstances and with special instruction, and it is likely to be especially useful for parents of infants who have repetitive febrile seizures.

- Tranxene (clorazepate dipotassium).

- Xanax (aprazolam).

Steroids

The corticosteroids (most people just say "steroids") are hormones made in the outer layer of the adrenal gland. They influence an incredible number of physical processes, including growth, organ function, and the body's response to stress. The steroids are also involved with regulating the immune system.

Steroids can help to stop certain types of severe seizure disorders in children and are sometimes used successfully by adults with epilepsy as well. How they do this is not understood. Steroids may work by provoking the body to produce additional hormones or other substances, by reducing inflammation in the brain, or by some other as yet unknown method.

Unfortunately, steroids also have serious side effects. You may have heard about "roid rage" (the technical term is corticosteroid psychosis), sudden aggressive outbursts that are known to occur in some athletes and body-builders who abuse illegal steroids. Steroids can cause sudden mood swings, making you irritable, depressed, and angry. They can also increase your appetite (leading to weight gain), raise your blood pressure and blood sugar levels, and lower the amount of potassium in your blood. In addition, taking steroids can suppress your body's immune response, leading to serious problems if you are inadvertently exposed to illnesses. Herpes viruses, including the common chickenpox virus, can be fatal to people taking high doses of steroid drugs. People who have tuberculosis, fungal infections, hepatitis B, and a wide variety of medical conditions require careful supervision while taking them. Corticosteroids may interfere with response to vaccines.

If your child needs a vaccine or any type of skin test (allergy, TB test), tell your child's doctor that she is taking steroids for her seizures.

Steroids interact with alcohol and other CNS depressants, including over-the-counter sleep aids, allergy and cold remedies that include ephedrine or other stimulants, and a long list of other medications, including Dilantin, blood-thinners, oral contraceptives, antibiotics, tranquilizers, and aspirin. If you are allergic to tartrazine dyes or sulfite preservatives, watch out—they are found in most steroid pills.

Luckily, when steroids are used to treat seizure disorders, it's usually on a short-term basis. With short-term use, the side effects disappear after treatment stops. Long-term steroid users, however, may develop early osteoporosis or joint damage called avascular necrosis. Discuss with your doctor whether calcium supplements are necessary.

Other hormones can also affect seizure disorders—the female hormone progesterone, for example, is believed to inhibit kindling. Although other types of hormones are not routinely prescribed to treat epilepsy at this time (except in clear cases of catamenial seizures, which increase just before the menstrual period begins), this is an area that a few researchers are investigating. It also helps to explain why the frequency and type of seizures often alters during periods of hormonal change, including puberty, menstruation, pregnancy, the post-partum period, and menopause. You may have noticed while reading the section on AEDs that many of them interact with oral contraceptives, an indicator that they do affect the hormone system in some way. There have been persistent reports over the years of patients whose seizures got markedly better or worse when taking contraceptives or hormones—not a reason to run out and ask for them, but a cause for interest and for caution when these drugs are prescribed.

Steroids are most commonly used to treat infantile spasms, Lennox-Gastaut syndrome, Landau-Kleffner syndrome, and myoclonic seizures. Prednisone (sold under many brand names, including Deltasone, Orasone, and Sterapred) and prednisolone (Prelone, Delta-Cortef) are probably the most commonly used steroids for epilepsy treatment.

Mysoline (primodone), also known as Apo-Primidone, Myidone, and Sertan, is another steroid sometimes used to treat forms of epilepsy. People with the disease porphyria, which is characterized by sensitivity to light, abdominal pain, and nerve damage, should not take Mysoline. If you have lung disease (including asthma), kidney disease, or liver disease, you will need to be carefully monitored while taking Mysoline. Take it with food to avoid nausea. Chewable tablets are available for children.

Adrenocorticotropic hormone (ACTH) is used to treat some types of seizures in children. It is given by injection. Some people are allergic to this medication, so a skin test should be done before the first injection. Parents, spouses, and caregivers can be taught how to give ACTH injections at home. Along with the behavioral effects noted earlier in this section, ACTH may cause fluid retention, and long-term use can cause nausea and slow growth in children. Overuse of ACTH may stimulate the adrenal gland too much, causing a serious condition known as Cushing's disease. Its symptoms can include mood swings, high blood pressure, excess growth of facial and body hair, weight gain, and reddening of the face and neck.

Notes about medications

Even the least powerful pill may be too much for some patients to start with. Some ways to take smaller doses of medications include:

- Medications taken in liquid form. Liquids can be measured out in tiny amounts, allowing for very gradual dosage increases. Children who refuse pills may take liquid medications readily. You can mix them with food or drinks (check with your pharmacist first). Be sure to shake the bottle well before pouring the medication, because the active ingredient may settle on the bottom of the bottle.

- Medications in capsule form that can be opened and divided into smaller doses, such as Depakote Sprinkles.

- Medications that can be broken into fractions. Pill splitters are available at most pharmacies for just this purpose. Make sure that it's okay to split a medication before you go this route, however: time-release medications and some pills with special coatings will not work properly when broken. Generally speaking, if the pill is scored down the middle, you can split it. If it isn't, ask your pharmacist or call the manufacturer's customer hotline.

- Medications that can be crushed and divided into equal parts. Some pills that are too small or too oddly shaped to split can be divided this way. Again, ask your pharmacist before doing this, as it's difficult to get precise doses with crushed pills. Tiny mortar and pestle sets can be found at health-food or cooking shops. You can buy empty gel caps to put the powder in, or you may be able to mix it into food or drink.

Compounding pharmacies make medications to order in their own labs. For example, they can make a liquid version of a prescription normally available in tablet form only, or a hypoallergenic version. If there isn't one where you live, you may be able to order over the Internet. Just use a search engine like AltaVista (*http://www.altavista.com*) or Lycos (*http://www.lycos.com*) to search for the term "compounding pharmacy." As always with Internet-based or mail-order businesses, check references before you pay for goods or services.

Giving medication to children can create special challenges. It is essential to get off to a good start and establish cooperation early. In the following suggestions from parents, you may find one technique that works well for your child.

> *To teach Brent (6 years old) to swallow pills, when we were eating corn for dinner I encouraged him to swallow one kernel whole. Luckily, it went right down and he got over his fear of pills.*

· · · · ·

> *I wanted Katy (3 years old) to feel like we were a team right from the first night. So I made a big deal out of tasting each of her medications and pronouncing it good. Thank goodness I tasted the prednisone first. It was nauseating—bitter, metallic, with a lingering aftertaste. I asked the nurse for some small gel caps, and packed them with the pills, which I had broken in half. I gave Katy her choice of drinks to take her pills with and taught her to swallow gel caps with a large sip of liquid.*

> *Gel caps come in many sizes. Number 4's are small enough for a three or four year old to swallow, but big enough to hold half of a 10 mg. prednisone tablet. Many other pills can be chewed or swallowed whole without taste problems. Just remember that children develop different taste preferences and aversions to medications, and gel caps are useful for any medication that bothers them.*

· · · · ·

> *After much trial and error with medications, Meagan's method became chewing up pills with chocolate chips. She's kept this up for the long haul.*

For younger children, many parents crush the pills in a small amount of pudding, applesauce, jam, frozen juice concentrate, or other favorite food.

> We used the liquid form of prednisone for my son, mixed it with a chocolate drink, and followed this with M&M's. The chocolate seemed to mask the taste.

> Whenever my son had to take a liquid medicine, such as antibiotics, he enjoyed taking it from a syringe. I would draw up the proper amount, and then he would put it in his mouth and push the plunger.

Teenagers' issues with taking pills are completely different from those for young children. The problems with teens revolve around autonomy, control, and feelings of invulnerability. It is normal for teenagers to be noncompliant, and they cannot be forced to take pills if they choose not to cooperate. Trying to coerce teens fuels conflict and tends to frustrate everyone. If you need help, ask for an assessment by a psychologist to work out a plan for adherence to treatment. Everyone will need to be flexible to reach a favorable outcome.

Lindy, mother of 15-year-old Joe, gives her view:

> I think the main problem with teens is making sure that they take the meds. Joe has been very responsible about taking his nightly pills. I've tried to make it easy for him by having an index card for the week, and he marks off the medicine as he takes it. I also put the meds on a dry erase board on the fridge as a reminder. As he takes the med, he erases it. That way it's easy for him (and me) to see at a glance if he's taken his stuff. The index card alone wasn't working because he couldn't find a pen, or forgot to mark it off.

> One of the biggest concerns with teens and maintenance is non-compliance. I think it's a delicate balancing act to allow teens to be responsible for taking their own meds and yet have some supervision of the process. Our meds are kept in a small plastic basket on the kitchen counter. All meds are taken there. I'd never want him to keep his meds in his room where I would have no idea if he had taken them or not.

> If he had shown any resistance to taking the meds, or any sign of telling me that he had taken them when he had not, I'd be doing this differently. My only other advice is to be sure to ask the doctors what to do

about a missed dose for each med. You are going to have a missed dose and it helps to know how to handle it.

Here are some more important do's and don'ts:

- Do not start or stop taking any prescription medication on your own, without first discussing it with your doctor.

- Be careful to follow dosage, time, and other instructions ("take with food," etc.) specifically.

- If you are pregnant or breastfeeding, or could become pregnant, ask your physician or pharmacist about any side effects specifically related to female reproduction and nursing.

- If you are actively trying to father a child, ask your doctor about male reproductive side effects.

- Tell both your physician and pharmacist about all other medications you take, including herbal remedies and over-the-counter drugs—even aspirin and cough syrup can cause dangerous side effects when mixed with the wrong medication.

- Avoid taking medications with grapefruit juice, which can prevent breakdown of certain medications.

- Inform your doctor about your use of alcohol, tobacco, any illegal drugs, and any vitamins or supplements (other than a regular daily multivitamin).

- If your doctor is unsure about how a medication might interact with a supplement, you may need to help her find more information about the chemical action of the supplement. Most doctors are not well-informed about nutritional supplements or herbal medicines, but many are willing to work with you on these matters.

- If you suspect that you have been given the wrong medication or the wrong dosage, call your pharmacist right away. Such errors do occur, and your pharmacist should be able to either reassure you or fix the problem.

You may find that there are occasions when your seizures become worse, and your regular maintenance medication and other strategies are not sufficient. For example, your seizures may tend to become worse just before your menstrual period or in times of great stress. Your doctor should be able to provide you with a small amount of medication to use on an as-needed basis for these times of unusually high seizure activity. This may be a few extra doses of your regular medication, or another prescription, such as an anti-anxiety drug like Ativan. Be sure that you understand when and how this medication should be used.

There may also be occasions when you need more help than your general practitioner or even your primary specialist can provide. Before you have a seizure-related crisis or need care when your doctor is unavailable, find out what facilities in your community offer the best urgent and emergency care for people with epilepsy. Your primary healthcare practitioner should be able to give you a list of recommendations.

Injections of medications like Valium can be given on an emergency basis to stop status epilepticus or severe seizures. The amount given is a much larger dose than would be used for regular seizure control, so this is almost always done in a hospital to prevent complications. Sometimes a parent, spouse, or caretaker can be trained to administer emergency medication if immediate access to a hospital is not available. For small children and infants, a rectal gel form of Valium is available and is easier to give at home.

Questions to ask your doctor

Prior to giving your child any drug or taking one yourself, you should be given basic information including answers to the following:

- What is the dosage? How many times a day should it be given?

- What are the common, and the rare, side effects?

- What should I do if side effects occur?

- Will the drug interact with any over-the-counter drugs, such as Alka-Seltzer or Tylenol? Will it interact with any herbal medicines or vitamins?

- Will I be given detailed counseling on avoiding risks such as drinking alcohol, smoking cigarettes or marijuana, and pregnancy?

- What should I do if I forget a dose?

- What are both the trade and generic names of the drug?

- Should I buy the generic version?

- Will this drug affect my vision, dental health, energy level, or sexual function? If so, are there remedies for these problems?

Prescription notes

You may see some odd initials on prescriptions or pill bottles. These stand for Latin words. Following are some of the most common abbreviations used by doctors and pharmacists:

Abbreviation	Latin Term	Meaning
ac	ante cibum	Take before meals
bid	bis in die	Take twice a day
gtt	guttae	Drops
pc	post cibum	Take after meals
po	per os	Take by mouth
prn	pro re nata	Take as needed
qd	quaque die	Take once a day
qh	quaque hora	Take every hour
qid	quater in die	Take four times a day
q(number)h	quaque (number) hora	Take every (number) of hours
q hs	quaque hora somni	Take at bedtime
q day	quaque day	Take once per day
tid	ter in die	Take three times a day
ut dict.	ut dictum	Take as directed

Drug interactions

Many people with seizure disorders also have other health problems. As you probably noticed when reading through the drug descriptions earlier in this chapter, AEDs interact with many other drugs, and these interactions are definitely a cause for concern. There are medications in almost every category (from pain medications used to treat arthritis to blood-thinners) that interact with AEDs. Many over-the-counter drugs, such as Tylenol or cough syrup, can also interfere with the medicines you take to control epilepsy.

Mixing AEDs and antidepressants or other psychiatric drugs is a particularly knotty area, especially for people with partial seizure disorders, who are more likely to need these medications. Both antidepressants and neuroleptics (antipsychotics), such as Haldol and Risperdal, lower the seizure threshold, and both affect and are affected by AEDs when they are taken together. The neuroleptics are very similar chemically to antihistamines, so if you take an AED that affects or is affected by antihistamines, this is a clue that it may also interact with neuroleptics. Generally speaking, AEDs will cause tricyclic antidepressants like Anafranil to last a shorter time, but tricyclics make AEDs last longer. Neuroleptic drugs leave the body quicker when you are also taking an AED, but they don't affect AED levels much at all. The newer SSRI antidepressants, such as Prozac and Luvox, can increase the amount of AEDs that reach the bloodstream. If you take a tranquilizer, such as Xanax, less of it will reach the bloodstream if you also take an AED.[4]

Drug interactions can make your AED more or less effective and can even lead to accidental overdose. Besides checking reference books and product literature for interaction warnings, one of the most important things you can do to avoid dangerous interactions is to get all your prescriptions filled at one pharmacy. Drug interactions are an area of special expertise for pharmacists. Many larger pharmacies have software installed that can automatically detect potential problems when you fill a new prescription.

Finally, check the contents of your pill bottle and its label each time you get a new medication or a refill. Sometimes dosage errors occur, and sometimes people are given the wrong medication, especially if your original prescription was scribbled or the drug you take has a name that's similar to that of another.

Beth tells how following this advice proved helpful:

> About a year ago I called in my prescription for one of the meds that I have been on for some time. I got home and started to put my tablets in the daily pill box when I noticed that the Depakote wasn't the right color—it was a darker orange. I called the pharmacist to see if the company had changed the pill in any way, and he replied that they hadn't. I then told him my concern, and he immediately offered to bring my prescription to my door. He had inadvertently given me the 500 mg pill instead of the 250 mg pill. I can only imagine how that would have made me feel in the morning.
>
> The only reason I had started to even pay attention to my meds was because of a special on PrimeTime Live. I looked at the prescription bottle and the info when I thought something was wrong, but it read as if it were 250 mg tabs. I'm glad I paid attention to my gut feeling on that.
>
> Ever since this happened, I check every med before I take it. I read the bottle and inspect the pills. What scares me is when meds are changed and you don't know what you're looking at.

Discontinuing medication

Never stop taking an AED, unless you are directed to do so by your doctor. Many people experience an increase in the number or severity of seizures ("seizure rebound") when they stop taking a medication suddenly.

Sometimes a doctor will ask that all medication be gradually withdrawn for a while to give her a baseline look at which symptoms are being caused by the disorder and which are due to over-, under-, or mis-medication. Also, you may need to stop taking one drug before starting another. This process can be exceptionally trying if it is not managed well. There are very few antiseizure medications that can be stopped cold without causing distress—and with some, this can be life-threatening.

Ask your doctor about symptoms to watch out for during the withdrawal period. She might be able to recommend over-the-counter or dietary remedies for likely problems, such as diarrhea or nausea. Decide in advance on non-medication strategies for dealing with seizures or side effects that may occur as your dosage is reduced.

Gradually tapering off to a lower dose and then to none is almost always the best approach. Medication changes should always be done under close medical supervision. In some cases (such as discontinuing benzodiazepine use after several years), medication withdrawal may need to take place in a hospital setting or under extra-careful home supervision.

Changing medications is sometimes nerve-wracking. Theresa, mother of Bryce, tells about their difficult experience with medications:

> Over the years, my son has taken every anticonvulsant drug available, either singly or in combination. He still has quite a few seizures every month. Recently, two new drugs were approved, and we wanted to see if either would be more effective in controlling his seizures. He was taking Topamax and Lamictal. We have started to slowly decrease the dose of Topamax. When he is off that, we will start him on a low dose of Trileptal.
>
> Every time we decrease one drug, his seizures get more frequent and stronger. He gets much more emotional with increased irritability and temper. If the seizures get really bad, I call the neurologist and ask to start the new drug early. The entire process—weaning off one and getting up to therapeutic doses of the replacement—takes about three months. It

exhausts the whole family. But we keep hoping for a drug that will really lessen or completely eliminate the seizures.

Blood tests and EKGs

Blood levels are a regular routine for people who take many AEDs. For example, liver or heart function may need to be tested before a particular drug can be tried, and perhaps at regular intervals during its use. Liver function is assessed with a blood test that checks the level of certain enzymes.

The insert that comes with your medication will include recommendations about how often you need blood tests, if at all. Experienced doctors have found that repeated blood tests are rarely needed on otherwise healthy patients whose medication is effective. If you have health problems that place you at special risk, such as heart or liver problems, regular blood tests become more important. Talk to your doctor about what kinds of tests she recommends when using your medication, how often you need the tests, and why they are necessary.

Other blood tests measure how much of the medication is found in the blood. Your doctor can compare this level to a chart of therapeutic blood levels: amounts of the medication that have been found to be effective in patients of various sizes and ages. The timing of blood draws can be important. Doctors usually aim for a trough level, meaning taking blood toward the end of a dose's presumed effectiveness. For example, if you normally take your medication at 8 a.m. and 5 p.m., late afternoon would be your best choice for having blood drawn for a trough level.

Theresa talks about her son's blood tests:

> *Bryce has taken every drug used to treat partial complex seizures. He first took Dilantin, and required fairly frequent blood tests until he achieved a stable level. With each subsequent drug, he seems to need fewer blood tests. Now, he gets them done every six to nine months. It seems that kids who find an effective medication have even less frequent blood tests.*

Always ask where your therapeutic blood level and current blood level are when you are tested. Observant patients can catch potentially dangerous mistakes. Typical problems include blood assessed with the wrong blood test, misinterpreted levels, and getting someone else's paperwork.

Once a therapeutic level has been reached, your main job is to try to keep that level steady. Sometimes this requires raising the dose of medication over time. It's as if the body gets used to the drug and requires more to get the same effect. This isn't the same as becoming addicted. Except for the benzo-diazepine tranquilizers, most of the drugs used to treat seizure disorders are not addictive when used as directed.

Good phlebotomists (blood-draw specialists) do not cause bruising or more than a twinge of pain when they do their job, unless you bruise very easily or have a low pain threshold. If this is the case, let the phlebotomist know—she may have a better way to obtain the sample. Numbing ointments (like EMLA cream) can help, although in some cases they cause the veins to constrict. You may have to experiment to find what works best for you.

People who do not have regular access to quality lab facilities, such as those living in remote areas, may have a very difficult time keeping up with a testing schedule. Talk to your healthcare provider about alternative ways to handle the need for monthly testing, such as having a visiting home-health nurse do the blood draw in your home and then mail the vial to a lab for testing.

Understanding blood test results

The results returned when you have blood test can be difficult to understand, unless you're a doctor. Here's some basic information about the three most common tests requested for patients taking AEDs:

- **Liver function tests.** The liver is the body's center for eliminating toxins, and since many AEDs include or produce toxins, they can put stress on the liver. Blood tests can be done that check the levels of liver (hepatic) enzymes. These enzymes result from the death of liver cells. Since the liver is constantly regenerating itself, some of these enzymes should always be present. What your doctor looks out for is an enzyme level that's much too high. The three liver enzymes most commonly checked are:

  - AST (aspartate aminotransferase), also known as SGOT (serum glutamic-oxaloacetic transaminase) or aspartate transaminase

  - ALT (alanine aminotransferase), also known as SGPT (serum glutamate pyruvate transaminase) or alanine transaminase

  - GGT (gamma glutamyl transpeptidase)

For people in good health, the levels of all three liver enzymes are usually below 25. Simply taking AEDs can double the level of liver enzymes. If the level goes over 70, that's generally considered cause for concern. If you have known liver problems or are experiencing health problems that could be caused by liver problems, your doctor might be concerned about levels between 35 and 70. High liver enzyme levels can also indicate heart problems.

- **WBC count.** WBC stands for white blood cells, also known as lymphocytes. A healthy number of white blood cells in your blood indicates a properly functioning immune system, a very elevated number can indicate the presence of infection, and a very low number can indicate either a suppressed immune system or an infection that has overwhelmed your body's defenses. The WBC count is included in a CBC count (see the following table).

- **CBC count.** CBC stands for complete blood cell, and as the name indicates, this test measures the numbers of various types of cells that should be present in your blood. It returns levels for both red and white blood cells, blood platelets, and subgroups of these cells. Typical, normal values returned from a CBC count are:

CBC Test Component	Expected Result
WBC (white blood cells)	5000–10000 WBCs per cubic millimeter of blood
HGB (hemoglobin)	12–15 grams per 100 cubic centimeters of blood
Hct (hematocrit)	31–43 percent of whole blood
RBC (red blood cells)	4–5.2 million RBCs per cubic millimeter of blood
Platelets	130,000–500,000 platelets per cubic millimeter of blood
MCV (mean corpuscular volume)	74–85, an expression of the average size of red blood cells

Normal CBC values for a specific person depend on that person's age, size, state of general health, and medications used. If one of your results on this or any other blood test seems to be outside the normal range, ask your doctor whether it should be a concern or not. Individual variations can occur and may not indicate a problem.

Drug level tests

Drug levels are especially important when you are in the process of changing medications or when you are using multiple medications. The efficiency of many, but not all, AEDs can be gauged with a blood test that measures the amount of medication present. Blood level testing is not always necessary, but when it is, a calendar can help you track dose changes in concert with blood levels and symptoms.

Chuck, husband to Kellie, explains:

> Kellie's transitioned through four meds (Neurontin, Tegretol, Topamax, and Dilantin) and is now on a combination of Lamictal and Keppra. Each time she's had to change meds, it's a long, drawn-out process where she has to scale back on one med, while ramping up on the other. Depending on the med and dosage, this can take anywhere from one to three months! Also during this process, Kellie is more prone to breakthrough seizures that occur when the med levels in her bloodstream get too low.

Electrocardiogram (EKG)

In addition to blood tests, your heart function may need to be monitored by regular blood-pressure tests, physical exams, and an electrocardiogram (EKG). The EKG can be done in the doctor's office, and since it uses wires that stick on the chest with an adhesive patch or gooey substance, it doesn't hurt at all. You just have to lie still (not always an easy task for kids). The wires are attached to a mechanical device or to a computer, much like an EEG machine, resulting in a graph of the electrical activity of the heart rate. Your doctor can read this graph to discern problems with or changes in heart function.

Vagus nerve stimulator

If you have tried seemingly everything when it comes to medication, with good medical supervision and medication trials of adequate length, your doctor may suggest a new treatment for epilepsy called the vagus nerve stimulator (VNS) or NeuroCybernetic Prosthesis (NCP). First approved for use in the US in 1997, this is a small, thin, disk-shaped device that is implanted in the chest. An electrical lead attached to the device runs under the skin to the vagus nerve in the left side of the neck. See Figure 5-1 for a representation in the body.

Like a heart pacemaker, the vagus nerve stimulator includes a special battery and a programmable computer chip. It is programmed to send controlled bursts of electricity to the left vagus nerve at regular intervals. Typically, these bursts last about 30 seconds and are sent every five minutes. This stimulation

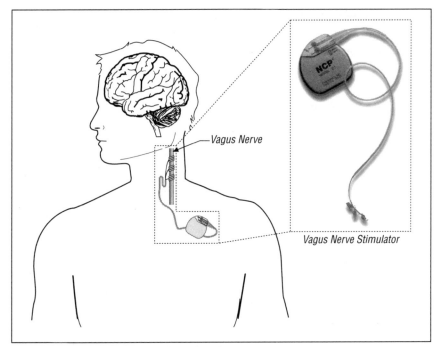

Figure 5-1. The vagus nerve stimulator (VNS)

has been shown to help prevent seizures in some people. If you experience an aura or other pre-seizure phenomena, you can use a magnet to activate and deactivate the device right away.

The vagus nerve stimulator does not work for all patients. It's also not generally a standalone solution. Most people who have one implanted continue to take AEDs.

Jill, parent of a child with multiple seizure types, explains:

> *My daughter had the VNS implanted seventeen months ago. By the ten-month anniversary we had noticed great improvements in her mood and outlook on life. Also, she was having fewer complex partial seizures, but they appeared more severe and lasted longer. During these seizures she often lost bladder control and tone in her legs, ending up on the floor. It had not made any difference with some other types of seizures (ESES). At this stage my daughter went nine days without a seizure—a rare event! The only change I made was about a month prior when I reduced her evening Topamax to 100mg (from 112.5) because she was having word-finding difficulties and was stuttering.*

Now, at the seventeen-month anniversary of the VNS implant and further gradual reduction in Topamax to 25mg BID, my daughter recently went eight weeks without a complex partial seizure until last week when she had two (less severe than previous ones and no loss of continence). She has not had an EEG recently so it is difficult to be certain whether the ESES has eased, but I feel it has because of the tremendous all-around improvements that she is showing. I hope the success continues!

Very, very few patients are lucky enough to become both seizure-free and drug-free thanks to the vagus nerve stimulator, but many are able to reduce their medication use and have an improved quality of life.

If you'd like to know more about the VNS, David Naess, a person with temporal lobe epilepsy who has a VNS, has created a superb introduction to the device at *http://www.howdydave.com/vns.html*. He discusses the cost, the implantation procedure, caring for the device after surgery, programming and activating it, and much more. It also includes photos of the device and associated accessories, and an excellent set of web links.

Surgery

Surgery is used only in rare instances as an option for treating epilepsy, but it can be both safe and effective for people whose seizures are not controlled on medication.

The journey toward surgery begins with reducing or discontinuing medications to permit a full and complete look at seizure activity. Brain imaging using MRI or CT scan is performed to gather more information. If brain abnormalities, a brain tumor, or areas of obvious brain damage are found during this process, these findings may make surgery imperative or rule it out as an option.

While this process is going on, the team should also delve deeply into the person's medical history to make sure that no treatment possibilities have been neglected. Sometimes at this point it's found that certain types of AEDs were never tried, that the person was not compliant with previous drug trials, or that there are other good reasons to avoid or delay surgery.

One factor that should not be allowed to rule out surgery is the presence of other handicapping conditions, such as mental retardation. Improved seizure control can greatly improve a person's quality of life, no matter what their IQ, life expectancy, or state of mental health.

Sometimes, invasive EEG testing (see Chapter 2 for information on this procedure) is necessary to pinpoint the exact location of the seizure focus. Video monitoring is done during the EEG, and the EEG is almost always done overnight or even longer.

Once a person has passed through the first preoperative phase, a second stage follows in which the focal area is determined. This includes neurological tests to figure out whether your left or right hemisphere is dominant, and the Wada test, in which Amytal (amobarbital, a central nervous system depressant) is injected into the internal carotid artery to put part of the brain to sleep. The person is monitored by EEG while the Amytal is active, and given more neuropsychological tests until the medication wears off. Depending on how the person responds to these tests, the doctor can figure out where in the brain speech and movement centers are located.

Finally, intracranial telemetry may be performed, meaning that electrodes are placed directly on the surface of the brain or even implanted deeper into the brain to pinpoint the focus (see the sections "Depth EEG" and "Subdural grid EEG" in Chapter 2 for more information).

If there is a small enough area involved in causing your seizures, the doctors may decide that you are a good candidate for surgery. The most typical area involved is the anterior temporal lobe and a deeper structure, the hippocampus. Up to 83 percent of patients who undergo an anterior temporal lobectomy—removal of part of these structures—eventually become seizure-free, although many still take medication after surgery. Others may experience a reduction in the number or severity of their seizures. A small number (between 1 and 2 percent) do not benefit.[5] If a different area of your brain is the focus, the success rate of the recommended procedure may be lower. Make sure that your neurosurgical team has ample experience with whatever procedure it is planning.

Jackie had a temporal lobectomy for her epilepsy in 1992 and was medication-free within two years. She shares her surgery experience:

> I went through a week of very strenuous testing to see if I was a candidate for surgery. It was miserable...I've never been through a sleep-deprived EEG before, so it was new to me and difficult. Then I spent all day in neuropsychological testing. They were intelligence tests—testing my knowledge and ability to think.

The doctor said I could be released after I had a SPECT scan. He said my seizures on the EEG were "beautiful," meaning they could tell where they were coming from—only one area of my brain. Two weeks later he called me to say they all agreed hands-down that I was a great candidate for surgery. They gave me a list that seemed fifty pages long of things that could "possibly" go wrong. Of course, death is always a possibility in any surgery. The only other ones that stick out in my mind are the possibility of losing my peripheral vision, and even more damaged memory.

It was my right temporal lobe that they were to remove. Before surgery, the right half of my head was shaved, from the center of my scalp all the way down. I was in surgery for six and a half hours. When I came out of it, I was purple, bruised, and very swollen. They had begun cutting about the center of my head along my hairline, cutting a backwards "C" (indenting only slightly) and ending the incision right in front of my right ear. I remained in the hospital for one week following surgery, taking great caution not to jar my swollen, sensitive brain.

I had been told to expect headaches non-stop after surgery, but I was hurting far worse than expected! I'd dealt with migraines for many years, but this was nothing in comparison. And for some reason, my jaw was killing me. I couldn't open my mouth wide enough to put a toothbrush in! It turned out that they had to remove part of my upper jawbone to get to my temporal lobe so they could get it out. I had to do jaw exercises for four months until it healed. Man, it was sore.

When I came home from the hospital, for one solid week there was to be no lifting, bending, cleaning, laundry, anything. I was confined to my bed or the couch (with brief visits to the potty)! My mother came to take care of my children. I have never felt such horrible head pains in my life. Childbirth may have been more painful, but it sure didn't last as many months as this did. I've got to say, recovery took just about a full year before I felt "back to normal" without the headaches.

Eight months after surgery, I got my driver's license back after going without it for thirteen years. By the end of the year, my neurologist told me I could try going off of my Tegretol anytime I desired. He casually said, "Come back and see me in a year, only if you need me." I never did. But I wrote him on November 30, 1999, letting him know it has been seven years and I'm still seizure-free, thanks to him.

New treatment possibilities

Many new treatment options are on the horizon. One area of emerging research is gene therapy, which is very, very experimental. Some researchers are working on new types of AEDs that can actually target specific genes, making them "turn off" the instructions that could be causing seizures. Other researchers are looking at the possibility of regenerating damaged areas that act as seizure foci using implanted stem cells, the master cells from which other cells evolve.

Taking off from today's VNS, even smaller devices could be created that target brain activity. One possibility that's under consideration is a miniature medication pump, much like the insulin pump now available for diabetes, that could deliver medication immediately when a linked sensor detects the start of a seizure.

Another device might send electronic stimulation to the substantia nigra, a brain region involved in some cases of refractory epilepsy. This kind of deep brain stimulation has been shown to help some patients with Parkinson's disease, and it might be especially helpful for children with partial complex seizures. Like the VNS, an electrode for deep brain stimulation is implanted during surgery and is attached to a pacemaker-like device implanted in the chest that can adjust the amount and type of stimulation.

Repetitive Transcranial Magnetic Stimulation (rTMS) is another promising area of research, and one that's non-invasive. Several studies have shown that low-frequency magnetic stimulation to the brain can help one-third or more of patients with refractory epilepsy, at least on a short-term basis. Don't confuse rTMS with the unscientific magnetic devices that have been peddled for years by various quacks. This is a treatment that, if it is eventually medically approved, would involve ongoing help from medical professionals. In fact, doctors testing rTMS must do a great deal of careful calibration before treating patients or risk causing unwanted effects and possibly even brain damage. If you'd like to delve into the literature on rTMS, the web site at *http://www.biomag.helsinki.fi/tms* is a great place to start.

Finally, immune-system research may help people who develop epilepsy as a result of brain infections or autoimmune activity in the brain. It appears that in some other cases of acquired epilepsy, a breakdown of the blood-brain barrier permits the formation of autoantibodies, including antibodies to brain tissue that could cause damage and then epilepsy. These antibodies attack brain tissue and can cause seizures.

Treatments geared toward these root causes may become available in the near future. Treating infections within the brain has not been easy in the past, but there have been a number of advances in this area recently. Researchers are experimenting with novel ways to deliver medication through the blood-brain barrier without opening the skull—for example, sneaking it in within a virus that has been genetically engineered to no longer cause disease.

Ongoing evaluation

Diagnosis should not be a one-shot affair, especially when the patient is a child. The gradual physical, emotional, and intellectual development of children can be affected by uncontrolled seizures. As your child matures emotionally, he will gain insight and skills that can help him take charge of his health, avoid known seizure triggers, and understand the importance of medication and other interventions.

Physical maturity matters too. Puberty in particular is a period of great upheaval, when symptoms can change drastically—for better or for worse. Try to ensure that your child is assessed at regular intervals for overall stability, response to medications, and adjustment to life. Both treatments and treatment goals will likely change as your child gets older. In periods of relative stability, for example, treatment may emphasize social, emotional, and academic development. You can take advantage of these periods to build skills that may make future episodes easier to handle. In periods of poor seizure control, goals may be much more basic.

Ongoing evaluation is also important for adults with seizures, of course, especially as you approach major milestones in life or when you are coping with new stresses. Pregnancy and childbirth, menopause, and aging are all times when seizure disorders may present new symptoms or become more or less difficult to treat and cope with. For more information about AEDs during pregnancy, childbirth, and breastfeeding, see Chapter 3, *Living with Partial Seizure Disorders*.

CHAPTER 6

Other Interventions

ALTHOUGH MEDICAL HELP is the key to seizure control, many people with epilepsy have found that diet and lifestyle changes, vitamins, supplements, and therapy are also useful. This chapter describes and evaluates the various possibilities.

Epilepsy treatment centers strongly encourage their clients to learn stress reduction techniques, to identify and avoid seizure triggers, and to use talk therapy as a way to work through some of the life problems that living with seizures can create. There's nothing unusual about any of these approaches; in fact, the most comprehensive programs provide such services on-site.

The ketogenic diet is also an accepted approach to treating refractory epilepsy in children. It is medically proven, but it must be carefully supervised by medical professionals.

Certain types of vitamin and mineral supplementation are often used to counteract medication side effects.

Other non-medication-based approaches to epilepsy do not enjoy the same degree of support among mainstream epileptologists. Some doctors are giving this area a second look, however, and most will support you in your quest for improved quality of life—as long as you don't go too far out on a limb or discard traditional approaches altogether. That said, many doctors (and especially neurologists, who are rather specialized) don't receive much training in alternative therapies. You will probably get the best results from working directly with a trained, licensed provider, such as a nutritionist or acupuncturist, who is willing to communicate and cooperate with your primary care provider.

It is very unwise to rely solely on non-medication measures to treat seizure disorders. There is much misinformation abroad in alternative healthcare circles. There is a potentially dangerous lack of scientific and regulatory supervision in this field, and sometimes a blatantly anti-science attitude as well.

Some alternative practitioners are well-trained and highly competent, while others are charlatans. Discussing all of your treatment options with your doctor and nutritionist will help you craft an individual treatment plan for your unique situation.

A holistic approach to epilepsy

The term holistic gets thrown around with abandon these days, even appearing in advertisements for shampoo and cosmetics. In healthcare, however, it has a very real meaning: considering all aspects of a person's physical, emotional, and spiritual well-being. It's an important concept when treating seizure disorders because of their far-reaching impact on people's lives.

Pat Murphy, a person with epilepsy and editor of the "Epilepsy Wellness Newsletter," puts it this way:

> *Stress is one of the leading causes for seizures, but the converse of that, as British epileptologist Dr. Peter Fenwick has said, is that "happiness is the best anticonvulsant." Experts say to look at what's making you stressed out. If you have a job you hate or problems with your spouse, or if you're poor, look at that and say, "Can I make some changes?"*

> *When you have epilepsy, you have this double whammy: doctors tell you that you have these defective neurons so the problem is within you, but the solution is without—take this drug. And along with medication come a lot of side effects, especially impaired concentration and fatigue. When I took phenobarbital years ago, I would feel so groggy when I woke up. Things would slip out of my hand for no reason at all.*

> *The other thing about drugs is they can take away symptoms, but they can't heal. If you take herbs, do biofeedback, acupuncture, whatever, you're healing your body and you feel better—and you feel like you have some control. I think that encourages you to take steps in other parts of your life as well.*

It's empowering to know that you can complement pharmaceuticals with other treatments, often reducing the dose and thereby eliminating some of their dangers and side effects. This combination approach is called complementary medicine: using the best of what medical science has to offer, and complementing it with supportive alternative practices.

A holistic view of epilepsy treatment is especially important for people with refractory seizure disorders. Don't give up on finding a better medication or combination of medications, but if it seems you have tried it all for an adequate amount of time without achieving adequate seizure control, you may find at least partial relief with a different approach.

Occasionally a person will have valid health reasons for giving up pharmaceutical treatments that are actually working. For example, almost all of the medications used to treat seizure disorders cause birth defects in a small percentage of infants born to women who need anticonvulsants. Pregnant and breastfeeding women who have epilepsy can find themselves faced with a terrible choice: compromise their own health or risk that of their child. Planning pregnancy in advance and temporarily relying on complementary methods under careful supervision (with a return to the use of effective medication as soon as possible) can help protect both the developing fetus and the mother's health. A person with epilepsy may also develop a serious health condition, such as cancer, that forces seizure medications to be temporarily discontinued during treatment. So even if complementary treatments are not right for you now, they might be useful someday.

Do not stop taking your AEDs without consulting your doctor. There is risk associated with stopping anticonvulsants and relying on complementary therapies; in particular, epileptic persons who stop their anticonvulsant medications sometimes develop status epilepticus—constant seizure activity. Status epilepticus may cause brain damage or death.

Complementary treatments rarely produce dramatic changes. When they work, they usually assist your body's own self-righting mechanisms, promoting better sleep, fewer and less severe seizures, improved general health, and a better frame of mind. Even when the benefits of vitamins or talk therapy turn out to be quite minor, the simple action of doing something on your own behalf is energizing and self-affirming—and you can't get that in a prescription bottle.

To get the clearest picture possible of the effects of complementary interventions, you should introduce them one at a time. Keep careful, daily records of supplements you introduce, when they are given and in what amounts, what brands you used, and any visible effects that you observe. If after four to six weeks you have not seen improvements with a supplement, it's unlikely that it will be of benefit. Dietary changes, talk therapy, and other interventions may take much longer to bear fruit.

Ask your primary epilepsy care doctor to make dietary changes, supplements, or talk therapy part of his prescription. Some doctors are very supportive, while others are not. Whatever you do, don't use complementary therapies behind your doctor's back—you need a medical expert on your team.

Environmental triggers

Adolescents and adults with seizures can often make lifestyle changes that reduce the number or severity of episodes. One of the most important of these changes is to become aware of environmental triggers. Avoiding discos with strobe lights, flickering fluorescent lights, TV commercials or shows that use strobe-like pulsing lights, poorly calibrated computer monitors that flicker, and certain types of carnival rides, for example, can be helpful. Learning relaxation techniques, such as meditation or biofeedback, may permit you to cope with triggers that can't be avoided entirely.

As Pat Murphy noted earlier in this chapter, perhaps the greatest environmental trigger of all is stress. Stress is a normal response to difficult life situations. It can be reduced but not avoided entirely. What can be changed is how you react to stress—with acceptance of the fact that things can't always go right, rather than with fear and worry. There hasn't been much hard research on stress reduction techniques that are especially appropriate for people with epilepsy, and what little research there has been is inconclusive. Still, anything that improves your general sense of control and well-being may help.

When you're feeling stressed out about a situation that has no immediate solution, such as an impending exam or work review, relaxation techniques can help defuse the tension. Perhaps the oldest relaxation methods around are meditation, prayer, and breathing exercises. These simple activities, either alone or in various combinations, relax the body and the mind simultaneously. There are many different schools of meditation and types of prayer or contemplative thought that have developed over the centuries and can fit any individual, of any religion (or none), in any situation. For instance, yoga offers many relaxation techniques that combine physical movements, special breathing patterns, and mental exercises. Working with a well-trained instructor can help you master whichever technique interests you most.

Breathing exercises can actually reduce the sensation of pain, gradually help agitation to subside, and even lower a racing heartbeat—as any woman who has tried Lamaze breathing during childbirth can tell you. One technique that works during anxiety or panic is sometimes called candle breathing. You breathe in through your nose in short breaths and breathe out gently through your mouth, as if blowing out a candle a couple of feet away. Done repeatedly, this usually has a calming effect.

Hyperventilation is a common side effect of extreme anxiety and panic. It can make a person pass out and can even mimic the physical sensation of a mild heart attack if you are unaware that you are hyperventilating. For people with seizure disorders, hyperventilation can trigger an episode. A hyperventilating person takes sharp, short, ragged breaths uncontrollably. Your whole body may seem to be wracked by the effort of this forced breathing. To stop the process, breathe into a small paper bag. As less oxygen comes in, your breathing process will slow down and become more regular until the episode of hyperventilation ends.

Hands-on relaxation techniques are especially effective for children. Parents report that slow, deliberate pressure on the head and joint compression (pressing together the knee and elbow joints from both directions) are calming activities for some, while others may respond better to more traditional massage. Occasionally a person with epilepsy will respond well to gentle chiropractic adjustments or other types of bodywork. Some people have reported benefits from EEG biofeedback, also known as neurofeedback. Be careful about "quack" providers in this area. Quite a few hospitals now offer neurobiofeedback programs, and these should be trustworthy.

Mary, age 57, who has temporal lobe epilepsy as the result of surgery to remove a brain tumor, says:

> Biofeedback is wonderful, very relaxing, and can really help with seizures. My neurologist says he knows of people that have used it with relaxation/visualization when they had the sense of seizures starting, and for some it even stopped their seizures. They learned how to do it through biofeedback.
>
> You are hooked up to a machine that's a lot like an EEG, except that you can see the display with your brain waves. My therapist plays soft music and uses wording to fit the situation, and I answer, for example:
>
> "Mary, do you prefer the ocean or the forest?"
>
> (Ocean.)

"What are you trying to overcome?"

(Seizures.)

"What do you find peaceful about the ocean?"

(The soft, gentle noise as it goes back and forth.)

"How do you visualize yourself on the ocean?"

(In a small boat, lying down, gently rocking back and forth, swaying, the sun flowing down on me.)

While this goes on we are measuring my pulse and heart rate, and how fast they go down.

As you gain mastery of the relaxation techniques used in neurobiofeedback, you can actually see the changes in your brain waves on the display. Once you have found visualization or other methods for calming your brain, you can call on these techniques when a seizure seems to be on its way.

Acupuncture and acupressure have also been shown to reduce self-reported stress levels for some people. Acupuncturists insert tiny needles just under the skin in areas believed to have a beneficial effect for your health condition; acupressure practitioners use pressure on similar points instead of needles. The method of action isn't understood, although Chinese medicine says it helps to redirect and harmonize the flow of energy in the body.

If you have allergies, you may find that your seizures increase during allergy season. This may be due to your body's production of its own natural antihistamines—or it could be caused by your antihistamine medication. Try to get your allergist and your primary care provider working together on a plan to reduce your allergies without using medication that lowers your seizure threshold. Positive steps might include lifestyle changes, such as adding an air filter to your bedroom or removing carpets that could harbor mold, combined with allergy shots or other forms of allergen desensitization.

Maintaining a consistent sleep schedule is also important for seizure prevention. Sleep deprivation is frequently a factor in seizures. Students, international travelers, shift workers, and others who may occasionally experience sleep schedule changes should consult their physician about medication changes and other techniques that may help them avoid seizures.

Seizure prevention

What do you do when you feel you have a seizure coming on? Many people with epilepsy have instinctively learned that lying down, dimming the lights, and relaxing can sometimes prevent or shorten a seizure. The same relaxation techniques that can reduce stress, including the use of positive imaging and biofeedback, can sometimes also work.

Certain odors are effective for "seizure-stopping," for some people and in some situations. In rural Iran, for example, pulling off your shoe and placing it under the nose of a person having a seizure is a popular folk remedy. The effectiveness of this technique is unknown, but it goes without saying that most people with epilepsy would not appreciate a whiff of stinky sneaker!

Researchers at the Birmingham University Seizure Clinic in the UK have explored the use of more pleasant forms of aromatherapy. Among the essential oils that appear to stop or reduce the severity of seizures for some people are lavender, chamomile, ylang ylang, jasmine, and bergamot.[1] Some other essential oils, notably rosemary and thyme, may have the opposite effect, and should be avoided.

Other people report that various types of touch are sometimes useful for stopping seizures, with useful interventions ranging from massage to tickling.[2] In China, acupuncture or acupressure is sometimes used. Ancient healers knew that compression, such as winding a sheet around a limb whose shaking often came before a seizure, sometimes worked.

You might try mild exercise (such as walking), listening to music that has either a calming or arousing effect, or nibbling on a food item. What works for you may be quite different than what works for someone else. In fact, it may not be the sensory experience or activity that stops the seizure, but the neurological processes that occur as a result of your belief that it will do so—a mental placebo effect, if you will, or a form of primitive biofeedback. What really matters is that these techniques often do work, and without causing harm. Once you have found a method for stopping or shortening at least some seizures, you will have gained just that much more control over epilepsy.

Counseling

Partial seizures can disrupt your life in many ways, particularly if you do not get adequate relief from medication. Some people have found that talking with a therapist can help. The focus of therapy is usually on understanding the condition, improving self-esteem, and talking about practical ways to handle difficult symptoms and situations. Many people with epilepsy rely on a trusted counselor or therapist when extra support is needed for decisions like revealing their medical condition at work, talking about epilepsy with a romantic prospect, or thinking about becoming a parent.

Children, and anyone who is newly diagnosed, benefit from having a knowledgeable person to talk to about their medical and personal concerns. Young people often suffer needlessly from fears related to their diagnosis but may be reluctant to talk to a parent about them. A good therapist knows what questions to ask and how to ask them.

The Epilepsy Foundation strongly recommends making family therapy part of the treatment plan for any child with epilepsy. This type of therapy is aimed at both education about the disorder and helping family members work together more effectively.

Of course, therapy is part of the regular treatment recommendations for mental conditions that may accompany partial seizure disorders, such as depression.

Your results will generally be best when working with a professional who understands the cognitive effects of seizures and AEDs. People who have seen therapists who are not knowledgeable about partial seizure disorders report that they must spend too much time explaining their diagnosis, and an inexperienced therapist may even try to second-guess it, attributing the effects of seizures to mental illness. No one needs that aggravation. If you can't find a local therapist who understands what you're going through, a self-help group may be a better source of support.

Theresa, mother of Bryce, says that therapy has been a good tool for her family:

> My son's seizure disorder is complicated by depression and learning
> disabilities. We have been to several therapists over the last eight years.
> What has made the biggest difference in his life was starting an antide-
> pressant. What has helped the family the most is finding a wonderful
> therapist. She helps me quite a bit on ways to handle my son's behavior,
> and this helps both him and me. She was also the first person who
> explained the neurospych test results in language I understood. Because
> she has counseled my son for years, she understands his complicated

brain functioning. She goes to all of our IEP meetings and explains to the committee what is really happening. She is our interpreter. She speaks their language, and that has been an enormous help in obtaining the services he needs. It bothers me to have to pay her to do what the school should be doing. However, without her support I'd be lost. For that reason, it's worth every penny.

Vitamins

A varied, healthy diet is your best source of vitamins. Some anti-epilepsy drugs (AEDs) can cause your body to metabolize certain vitamins differently, and therefore some people who take them require carefully planned diets or supplementation. For most people, a daily multivitamin supplement addresses any deficiency that may occur from missing your veggies on occasion.

Some people swear that vitamins prevent or weaken seizures and counteract certain medication side effects. Vitamins certainly can influence epileptic activity, and they can also affect and be affected by AEDs. Although vitamin supplementation has a long history as a complementary therapy for epilepsy, there is no medically proven way to prevent seizures using vitamins alone—except in the case of using B6 for a specific type of infantile seizures.

If you plan to pursue vitamin therapies, buy a basic guide to vitamins and minerals that includes information about toxicity symptoms. Some people metabolize vitamins and minerals differently and may be more or less susceptible to potential toxic effects. Along with your doctor's guidance, a good reference book can help you avoid problems. See Appendix A, *Resources*, for some suggestions. Also, take vitamin company sales pitches and dosage recommendations with a grain of salt. The testimonials these companies produce are intended to sell their products, not to help you develop a treatment plan. Consult a physician or a professional nutritionist who does not sell supplements for unbiased, individualized advice.

The vitamins used most often to control seizures or AED side effects follow.

Vitamin B3

Vitamin B3 (niacin) has anti-inflammatory qualities and helps to build and rebuild nerve tissue. It's also needed when the body synthesizes its own fatty acids and corticosteroids. People who take AEDs must be careful about niacin, however, as it can intensify the effects of some medications. This fact could be used to the advantage of those who are trying to reduce their AED dose for side effect prevention, although deliberately potentiating an AED with niacin must be done under medical supervision.

Vitamin B6

Seizures in infants are sometimes caused by vitamin B6 deficiency and may be successfully treated using oral or intravenous vitamin B6. Its usefulness for other people who have seizures is unsubstantiated, but case reports of such seizure prevention benefits in older children and adults are common.

What is known is that B6 is essential for metabolism of amino acids, proteins, fatty acids, and starches, and for the production and proper use of neurotransmitters. B6 binds to the same receptors as natural corticosteroids, and may regulate steroid production by this mechanism.

Depakote (valproic acid) appears to deplete B6, and other AEDs may affect how the body uses this vitamin as well. Adding B6 when you are taking an AED may actually make your medication work better—but this must be done under medical supervision. B6 must be given with magnesium to ensure absorption. Ask your doctor about the appropriate amount of each to use.

Most people should avoid "megadoses" of vitamins. However, high doses of B6 are sometimes recommended for people with epilepsy or related neurological conditions, and there is solid evidence that they are both safe and effective for some persons.

If you experience agitation or tingling of the hands or feet while taking B6, reduce your dose until these symptoms disappear.

Vitamin C

While it hasn't been shown to cure the common cold, vitamin C is certainly helpful for promoting good general health. More importantly for people with epilepsy, it acts as an antioxidant, which may help to protect your body from the harmful effects of AEDs, and which is needed by the body for synthesis of neurotransmitters, natural corticosteroids, and carnitine.

Vitamin D

AEDs seem to affect how the body metabolizes vitamin D, which can in turn affect calcium levels. The end result can be loss of bone tissue (osteomalacia). Getting out in the sunshine should provide you with plenty of vitamin D, as the body can usually produce its own supply if you get enough sun. However, if tests show that you are already experiencing osteomalacia or osteoporosis, taking both vitamin D and calcium supplements may help.

Vitamin E

Vitamin E does appear to have antiseizure properties. In one study of refractory epilepsy in children, 10 of 12 persons experienced a significant reduction in seizures while taking 400 mg of E daily.[3]

If you experience skin or hair problems due to AED use, supplementing with vitamin E may help. This fat-soluble vitamin also offers some protection against tardive dyskensia, a serious and permanent movement disorder associated with some psychiatric drugs.

Vitamin K

"Vitamin K" is actually a group of vitamins that have been lumped together under one name. They are essential for liver function and blood clotting, among other things. When pregnant women take AEDs, their offspring may be deficient in vitamin K, leading to serious bleeding disorders. A 10 to 20 mg per day dose is the current recommendation for women who are or could become pregnant.[4]

Other people with epilepsy probably do not need to worry much about vitamin K. However, a small supplementary dose may be a good idea for people taking AEDs that are processed by the liver, especially people with impaired liver function.

Folic acid

Folic acid is a water-soluble vitamin that helps make the rest of the B vitamins available to the body. It builds and repairs the nervous system and acts as an anti-inflammatory. Folic acid appears to reduce the frequency of seizures for most people and may allow some to reduce their AED dose as a result.[5] However, a few people have more seizures on quite low doses of this supplement.[6]

Folic acid absorption is affected by several AEDs, including valproic acid (Depakote), carbamazepine (Tegretol), and phenytoin (Dilantin). Dilantin apparently competes with folic acid in the gastrointestinal (GI) tract and brain. Accordingly, if you take an AED, talk to your doctor about whether you need or should avoid extra folic acid, especially if you are or could become pregnant. Lack of folic acid is especially dangerous during pregnancy, when it can cause neural tube birth defects and can also contribute to heart disease and other health problems. Supplementing with small amounts of folic acid (1 mg or less) is now recommended for all women who are or plan to become pregnant.

Biotin

Biotin helps the body produce fatty acids, and it is needed for metabolism of proteins and other B vitamins.[7,8] Some AEDs deplete or interfere with this little-known but important relative of the B vitamins.

Minerals

Minerals are naturally occurring substances and are basic building blocks for cells and chemical processes in the body. Most of them are needed in such small amounts that the average person's needs are easily covered with a reasonably decent diet and a regular multivitamin with minerals. However, some minerals are needed with the extra vitamins that some people taking AEDs require, and others can help reduce common AED side effects. The following sections describe minerals that are sometimes suggested.

Calcium

Calcium can help prevent bone loss, which is associated with long-term use of some AEDs and steroids. It's also important for the regulation of impulses in the nervous system and for neurotransmitter production. If you supplement with magnesium, you should also take twice that amount of calcium—these two minerals need each other to work. However, excessive levels of calcium (hypocalcinuria) can cause stupor.

Chromium picolinate

Chromium picolinate may help control the sugar and carbohydrate cravings that many people experience while taking Depakote or Depakene. Chromium picolinate can act like a stimulant in some people, and thus may also counteract AED-induced fatigue.

Magnesium

Magnesium lowers blood pressure and is also important for the regulation of impulses in the nervous system and neurotransmitter production. Magnesium deficiency can cause anxiety and insomnia, and it can also lower your seizure threshold. This mineral is rapidly depleted during periods of stress, hard work, hot weather, or fever, and that's probably one of the reasons that these conditions can precipitate a seizure. If you are supplementing with vitamin B6, you will need to add magnesium as well. Magnesium also blocks calcium channels and dilates blood vessels, so watch out for interactions with medications that have similar or opposite actions.

Manganese

Deficiency of manganese is marked by fatigue, irritability, memory problems, and ringing or other noises in the ears. Some of the problems attributed to manganese deficiency are also known side effects of certain AEDs, and there could be a relationship—but only trace amounts of this mineral are needed. The amount of manganese included in a typical daily combined vitamin and mineral supplement (usually 2.5 to 5 mg) should be sufficient.

Zinc

Zinc is another trace mineral that's often absent from the diet. Symptoms of deficiency can include mental disturbance. If you have GI tract problems due to celiac disease or stomach irritation from your medication, a little extra zinc might be helpful. The recommended dose is 15 to 20 mg of the chelated form of zinc (5 to 10 mg suffices for children).

Supplements

If it's not an herb, vitamin, or mineral, additions to the diet are called nutritional supplements. That means the manufacturer agrees not to market it as a drug, and the FDA agrees to consider it a food. Meanwhile, consumers are left unsure about whether these supplements provide nutrients (they usually don't), cure disease (rarely, if ever), or simply promote health. In addition, new anticonvulsant medications become available in the United States only when they are shown to be safe and effective using good quality scientific studies (prospective double-blinded studies). Complementary medications are sold in the US even though they may have not met this same high standard of safety and effectiveness.

The following is a list of supplements that may be suggested to people with seizure disorders:

- **Carnitine.** Also known as beta-hydroxy-gamma-trimethylammonium butyrate, carnitine is a substance that helps long-chain fatty acids get through the inner membrane of mitochondria within individual cells. It is depleted by use of Depakote and similar drugs. Symptoms of very low carnitine levels may include fatigue, jaundice, nausea, and confusion, and the condition can be associated with liver damage.[9,10] Carnitine levels can be tested, and supplements are available by prescription.

- **Choline.** One of the active ingredients in lecithin (see later in this list) is choline. The brain needs it for processes related to memory, learning, and mental alertness, as well as for the manufacture of cell membranes and the neurotransmitter acetylcholine. It appears to be involved in emotional control and other regulatory functions, but its effectiveness for seizure control is unknown.

- **GABA.** Gamma aminobutyric acid is an amino acid–like compound that inhibits the activity of other neurotransmitters. It is definitely involved in seizure suppression, but that may be a good reason not to take it— you might be getting yourself into real trouble. Gabapentin and Depakote are among the AEDs that affect the brain's own GABA production or use. You should never take these medications with GABA supplements, unless your physician recommends it and oversees the process. Supplementation with over-the-counter GABA is sometimes recommended for anxiety, nervous tension, and insomnia, especially insomnia associated with racing thoughts. If you experience shortness of breath, tingling, or numbness in your hands or feet when taking GABA, lower or discontinue this supplement.

- **Inositol.** Inositol is one of the active ingredients in lecithin (see later in this list). It is required by the neurotransmitters serotonin and acetylcholine, and it may repair some types of nerve damage. Clinical studies indicate that inositol supplements may be helpful for some people with obsessive-compulsive disorder, depression, and panic disorder. Its effectiveness for seizure disorders is unknown.

- Lecithin. Also known as phosphatidyl choline, lecithin is a phospholipid found mostly in high-fat foods. It is said to have the ability to improve memory and brain processes, although double-blind studies of people with Alzheimer's disease did not substantiate claims that it can help people recover lost brain function. The ketogenic diet increases the amount of lecithin in the body, which may be one of the reasons for its success. Some people with epilepsy have also reported that their number and severity of seizures was reduced from taking lecithin alone. Lecithin capsules are available, but many people prefer the soft lecithin granules. These are a nice addition to fruit-juice smoothies, adding a thicker texture. Lecithin is oil-based, and it gets rancid easily. It should be refrigerated.

- Melatonin. This sleep-regulation hormone is produced by the pineal gland. The amount of melatonin in the body is reduced by nighttime doses of valproic acid and may be affected by other AEDs.[11] One way to deal with this problem, should sleep disruption be the result, is taking a melatonin supplement before going to bed. Supplementing directly with any kind of hormone can be problematic in the long run, however, as your body might respond by producing less of the natural substance. If you're considering melatonin, talk about it with your doctor, and set up a dosage plan and observation schedule.

- Taurine. This amino acid appears to have antiseizure capabilities. It inhibits abnormal electrical activity in the brain and is often deficient in brain tissue where seizures have been occurring. Recommendations range from 500 to 1000 mg per day, divided into as many as three doses. Experts recommend buying only pharmaceutical-quality L-taurine from reputable manufacturers. Unusual EEG activity has been reported in people using doses over 1000 mg per day.

- Tyrosine. Another amino acid, tyrosine serves as a precursor to the neurotransmitters norepinephrine and dopamine. It may help the body form more of these neurotransmitters, and it is also believed to provide support for optimal thyroid gland function. Tyrosine can raise blood pressure, so talk to your doctor about using it if you take other medications that affect blood pressure.

- **Phenylalanine.** This is an essential amino acid, as well as the precursor of tyrosine (see earlier in this list). Like tyrosine, phenylalanine can raise blood pressure.

- **SAMe.** S-adenosyl-methionine is a metabolite of methionine that is used in Europe to treat depression and arthritis. It became available in the US in early 1999. It is believed to affect dopamine and serotonin, and to have anti-inflammatory effects. It may affect serotonin so talk to your doctor before taking this along with an AED.

Herbal remedies

Before chemical anticonvulsants were concocted in the lab, people with epilepsy around the world relied on herbal medicines known as nervines. As the name indicates, these are herbs that affect the nervous system.

If an herbal remedy has gained a reputation as a nervine, it is likely to have actions in your body similar to those of a prescription drug. You should use the same degree of caution with herbal remedies as you would with their chemical cousins, some of which are actually based on chemicals first derived from herbal remedies. Some nervines may have mild antiseizure qualities, some are sedatives that can affect you like a dose of Valium, and others combine various actions.

No double-blind clinical trials in the US have evaluated the effect of herbs on seizure activity. There have been many clinical trials of herbal formulas in Europe, however, and standardized herbal remedies are available by prescription and are widely used in Germany. However, you must still research carefully and proceed with caution, especially if you are planning to use an herbal remedy at the same time as a prescription drug.

Another problem with herbal remedies is reliability, especially in the US, where they are unregulated. Botanical formulas can differ wildly in their potency, both from manufacturer to manufacturer, and from vial to vial. Consistent dosing is imperative for seizure control and to avoid interactions with prescription drugs, so the problem of ensuring the same dosage strength and size is a concern.

Cautions aside, the topic of herbal remedies is always of interest. Some traditional nervines follow, gathered from a variety of herbal manuals old and new:

- Black cohosh (*Cimicifuga racemosa*). This nervous system depressant and sedative may also have anti-inflammatory effects. Its active ingredient appears to bind to estrogen receptor sites, so it may affect hormonal activity.

- Black currant (*Ribes nigrum*). This berry has been used as an anti-inflammatory.

- Chamomile (*Anthemis nobilis*). Chamomile is a mild but effective sedative traditionally used to treat sleep disorders or stomach upsets. It is a member of the daisy family, so avoid this herb if you are allergic to its cousin, ragweed.

- Damiana (*Turnera aphrodisiaca*). This is a traditional remedy for depression. As its Latin name indicates, it is also believed to have aphrodisiac properties. Its energizing quality might not be desirable for people who tend to get agitated, but a few doctors recommend it to counter the libido-deadening effects of some types of seizures and certain AEDs.

- Gingko biloba. An extract of the gingko tree, gingko biloba is advertised as an herb that can improve your memory. There is some clinical evidence for this claim. It is an antioxidant and is prescribed in Germany for treatment of dementia. It is believed to increase blood flow to the brain.

- Grapeseed oil and Pycogenol. Both grapeseed oil and Pycogenol (which is derived from marine pine trees) are powerful antioxidants. Some people take them to prevent toxic effects of medications; others claim that they have a calming effect on behavior and activity level.

- Gotu kola (*Centella asiatica, Hydrocotyl asiatica*). Gotu kola is an Ayurvedic herbal stimulant sometimes recommended for depression and anxiety.

- Hops (*Humulus lupulus*). Hops is the herb used to flavor beer and the reason beer makes many people sleepy. It's available in capsules or as a dried herb for use in tea, and it works as a gentle sleep aid.

- Kava-kava (*Piper methysticum*). This mild sedative herb has been used for centuries in the South Pacific. A member of the pepper family, kava-kava appears to have benzodiazepine-like effects on anxiety—but without causing sedation and mental dulling. It is believed to work primarily within the limbic system. Some people develop a skin rash when taking kava-kava and should avoid this herb thereafter.[12]

- Licorice (*Glycyrrhiza glabra, Liquiritia officinalis*). Licorice boosts hormone production, including hormones active in the digestive tract and brain. This is related to, but not the same as, the herb used to flavor sweet licorice.

- Mistletoe (*Viscum album*). Mistletoe has narcotic and antispasmodic qualities and has been used to treat epilepsy since ancient times. It figured prominently in the remedy lists of 16th and 17th century physicians in Europe. Its mode of action is probably similar to that of the benzodiazepine tranquilizers, including causing sedation and lethargy.

- Passion flower (*Passiflora incarnata*). This flower has sedative, antispasmodic, and anti-inflammatory qualities. Along with skullcap and mistletoe, it was probably the Western herb most frequently used to treat epilepsy before pharmaceutical AEDs were invented.

- Sarsaparilla (*Hemidesmus indicus*). Like licorice, sarsaparilla seems to affect hormone production and also settle the stomach and calm the nerves. If you try sarsaparilla, make sure you get the correct variety. The name is sometimes used in the US for a different type of plant that is related to ginseng.

- Skullcap (*Scutellaria lateriflora*). Skullcap is a medium-strength sedative with anticonvulsive properties. Traditional uses include menstrual irregularity and breast pain, indicating that it probably has hormonal effects.

- St. John's wort (*Hypericum perforatum*). This plant has gained popularity as an herbal antidepressant. It has the backing of a decent amount of research, but those choosing to use this remedy should follow the same precautions as with SSRIs and MAOIs, two families of pharmaceutical antidepressants. It can cause increased sensitivity to light. It is available by prescription in Germany, where it is the most widely used antidepressant. It is potentially dangerous to use St. John's wort with any other medication that could affect serotonin, a category that includes many AEDs. It may also decrease the effectiveness of birth control pills and counter protease inhibitors and certain medications used by organ transplant recipients.

- Valerian (*Valeriana officinalis*). This is a strong herbal sedative (and one of the ingredients in the soporific liqueur Jagermeister). It should not be given to young children.

In addition to these European and American herbs, there's an entire pharmacy of Asian herbal remedies, including those found in India's Ayurvedic medicine and various types of Oriental herbology. Using these systems of medicine properly requires working closely with an experienced, qualified practitioner, not buying something off the shelf. Usually herbs are used only as part of a complete health-promotion program involving diet, meditation, and other therapies.

Both the Ayurvedic and Oriental systems pre-date Western medicine by some hundreds of years, and no doubt both have discovered some useful treatments. However, some Chinese herbal remedies in particular are very strong, often relying heavily on stimulants like Ma Huang (ephedra) and ginseng to give people a quick pick-me-up. Neither system has found a cure for epilepsy, although occasionally overly ambitious practitioners will advertise one. Use great caution with all herbal remedies.

Essential fatty acids

Essential fatty acids (EFAs) are compounds needed to build cells and also to support the body's anti-inflammatory response. They are the "good" polyunsaturated fats that improve cardiovascular health when substituted for the "bad" saturated fats. More importantly for people with epilepsy, they appear to have some effect on neural functioning, preventing misfires and possibly short-circuiting the kindling process. There's a great deal of medical research going on in this area, particularly on the efficacy of EFAs as a treatment for bipolar disorders.

There are two major types of EFAs, Omega-3 and Omega-6. Two Omega-3 fatty acids are found in oily, cold-water fish: eicosapentaenoic acid (EPA) and docosahexanoic acid (DHA). Another Omega-3 fatty acid, alpha-linoleic acid, is found in flaxseed and perilla oils, among other sources. The Omega-6 family includes linoleic acid and its derivatives, including gammalinolenic acid (GLA), dihomogamma-linolenic acid (DGLA), and arachidonic acid (AA). These substances also come from animal fats and some plants, such as evening primrose oil (EPO), which is a good source of GLA, flaxseed oil, black-current seed oil, hemp-seed oil, and borage oil, which contains both GLA and very long chain fatty acids (VLCFAs).

Unfortunately, the high levels of arachidonic acid found in evening primrose oil have been reported to lower the threshold for frontal-lobe seizures, so people with epilepsy should exercise caution. Also, the VLCFAs found in borage oil can be irritating to the liver and central nervous system and are therefore not recommended for use by children and people with nervous-system disorders, or for people taking AEDs that put a heavy load on the liver. Other oils with a high VLCFA content are canola oil, peanut oil (including the oil in peanut butter), and mustard-seed oil.

When oils are heated, most will convert at least part of their fatty acids into trans-fatty acids, which are substances to be avoided. Hemp oil is one of the few that can resist this heat-driven conversion progress, and it has recently become available for cooking and medicinal use in the US. Researchers believe that achieving a dietary balance between Omega-3 and Omega-6 fatty acids provides the most benefits. The ratios usually recommended are 3:1 or 4:1 Omega-6 to Omega-3.[13]

EFA basics

Now that you know the good news about EFAs, here's the not-so-good news: in the much-touted McLean Hospital study in which people with bipolar disorder successfully prevented kindling episodes with EFA supplements, participants took 9.6 grams per day of concentrated fish oil. Think about that for a moment: 9.6 grams is a lot of oil to drink from a spoon, much less take in capsule form (that's almost 30 capsules per day). Many persons who have tried to duplicate this experiment at home have found it difficult, both for the sheer amount they had to use and for the side effects that can ensue.[14]

Since announcing his initial results, McLean researcher Dr. Andrew Stoll has produced a "Omega-3 Fatty Acid User Guide."[15] He notes that five grams of Omega-3 fatty acids may be sufficient to stabilize mood in adults (of course, the dose for children should be reduced according to body weight). Although he recommends fish oil because it has been studied the most, Dr. Stoll notes that the concentration of Omega-3 EFAs in flaxseed and perilla oils is actually higher, and the taste of these oils is far more palatable (however, he does not recommend flaxseed oil to persons with bipolar disorder, because some people in a his study group became manic while taking it). Two to three teaspoons per day of these oils in their liquid form should be sufficient for an adult, he says, although dosage will need to be adjusted according to body size and individual chemistry. Dosage for children will depend on size and weight. The maximum effective dose Dr. Stoll reports using for adults is 15 grams of oil per day.

What does this all mean for people whose problem is seizures, not mood swings? Well, assuming that there is a basic similarity between the kindling processes in manic-depression and in epilepsy, it's quite possible that EFAs could help some people achieve better seizure control. The doses used might be different, but right now Dr. Stoll's guide is the only professional data available.

EFA tips

The following tips for using EFAs have been collected from a variety of sources, including researchers at NIH, US mood disorder clinics that are trying this approach, and people with epilepsy themselves:

- Take antioxidant supplements during treatment with EFAs, to prevent your body from simply oxidizing the extra oil. One mood disorder clinic recommends 1200 IUs (International Units) of natural vitamin E and 2000 mg of vitamin C for adults weighing approximately 150 pounds, with doses for children reduced according to body weight.

- If you choose fish oil, "fishy burps" are the most commonly reported side effect—and they are most unpleasant. Some people recommend swallowing a whole clove of garlic or a garlic tablet with the fish oil as a "breath deodorant." You know these burps are not nice if garlic is recommended as a cover-up! Taking the fish oil at night or with orange juice also seems to help.

- In Iceland and Scandinavia, flavored fish oils have long been available as an old-fashioned health tonic (mint is a favorite). If demand rises, these may be seen on North American shelves soon. If you're curious about these, see *http://www.lysi.is/wpp/lysi/lysi.nsf/pages/contents*.

- Stomach troubles and excessive flatulence may result from EFA use. Garlic or a garlic pill might help with these problems. Some people report trying acidophilus capsules or other probiotics, yogurt with live cultures, or over-the-counter stomach or gas remedies. If you try OTC medications, do be careful. Many of these can interact with or counteract psychiatric medications, and they just might affect the action of EFAs as well. Perilla oil seems to be better tolerated by the stomach than fish oil or flaxseed oil.

- Diarrhea or oily stools can be another unpleasant side effect, especially if the dose is over ten grams per day. In fact, flax seeds are well-known for promoting regularity, and if you ingest a lot, you may get diarrhea. Taking several small doses of oil rather than one large one should help.

- Make sure your oil has been toxicology tested and prepared and stored to prevent it from being rancid. The presence of mercury in the liver tissue of some large ocean fish has led some fatty-acid researchers to warn consumers about using untested cod liver oil, and to recommend using oil prepared from fish skin instead. Plant-based oils could also contain pesticide residues, unless they are certified as organic. Toxicology-tested fish oils are available from several sources, however, including Kirkman Labs (800-245-8282, *http://www.kirkmanlabs.com*) and OmegaBrite (512-288-2700).

It's great if you can get at least some of your EFAs in food. Low-fat diets are part of the reason some people, especially those who are trying to lose weight, may not get enough. Many cold-pressed salad oils, including olive, safflower, sunflower, corn, peanut, and canola oils, do contain EFAs, as do coconut oil and coconut butter. When these oils are processed with heat, however, the fatty acids may be changed or destroyed. Corn and soybean oils are both rather high in Omega-6 fatty acids. Olive oil is probably your best EFA-rich choice for oil-based dressings and marinades.

Oily, cold-water fish themselves are another great EFA source, although again, the Omega-3s are affected by cooking (and not everyone is a sushi fan).

It is possible to have lab tests done to discern EFA levels, although these are rarely ordered. You might have your doctor send a blood sample to a lab that specializes in this type of test.

Diabetics may experience adverse effects from too much of certain EFAs, either in the diet or in supplement form, and should talk to their physician before making EFA changes. If excess weight is already a problem for you, you should consult a nutritionist about how to substitute these good fats for bad, while cutting calories in other areas.

Some commercial EFA preparations follow.

- **Efalex.** This brand-name EFA supplement made by Efamol Neutriceuticals, Inc., is widely touted as a supplement for people with ADD/ADHD. It contains a mix of Omega-3 fish oil, Omega-6 evening primrose oil and thyme oil, and vitamin E. Another product from the same firm, Efamol, is marketed as a treatment for PMS. It combines evening primrose oil; vitamins B6, C, and E; and niacin, zinc, and magnesium. Both products are now available in the US, Canada, and the UK, and they can be purchased by mail order. Unlike many supplement manufacturers, Efamol adheres to strict standards and also sponsors reputable research. However, note that both of these products include evening primrose oil, and make your decision accordingly.

- **EicoPro.** Made by Eicotech, Inc., this product combines Omega-3 fish oils and Omega-6 linoleic acid. Eicotech is another supplement manufacturer known for its high manufacturing standards.

- **NutriVene-D.** This supplement, created especially for people with Down's syndrome, mixes EFAs, vitamins, and other substances.

- **Essential Balance/Essential Balance Jr.** This EFA supplement is made from sesame, sunflower, flaxseed, pumpkin-seed, and borage oils. The adult formulation is a capsule, while the children's version is available as a liquid.

Diet

If you suspect that certain foods trigger your seizures, it's fairly simple to eliminate them from your diet one at a time to see what happens. If you think that major changes may be needed, however, the best practitioner to see is a qualified nutritionist.

Robert explains how food intake affects his complex partial seizures:

> My neurologist has diagnosed me as having what he calls "complex reflex epilepsy," which merely indicates that my seizures are triggered. In my case, most of my seizures occur during meals. Checks have been done for "dumping," an unfortunate term used to describe the stomach contents rapidly emptying, raising blood sugar. My seizures last typically less than a minute, though occasionally longer.

> My epilepsy started with nocturnal grand mal seizures 23 years ago, which were successfully controlled for about fifteen years. Since I had chemotherapy, my complex partials have remained uncontrolled, despite trying all the AEDs except Tegretol, which may dangerously affect an already low white blood count.

Nutritionists are experts in how food intake affects health. Hospitals, clinics, and long-term care facilities employ nutritionists to improve patient care through appropriate diet. Others work in private practice. Some nutritionists have very traditional views about diet, while others may recommend what seem like radical changes. Be sure to check the credentials and training of any nutritionist you consult.

As the previous section on essential fatty acids indicated, one dietary change that may help is eliminating most hydrogenated (trans) fats. Experts in fatty acid metabolization note that hydrogenated fats short-circuit the body's ability to metabolize the good fatty acids needed to produce normal amounts of neurotransmitters and other hormones, and to protect and calm the nervous system.

Some nutritionists recommend that people with seizure disorders also avoid the protein-based artificial sweetener aspartame (NutraSweet). One study showed an increase in absence seizures in children who drank soft drinks containing aspartame.[16]

Alcohol is also an item to avoid or at least use with moderation. It is often a contributing factor to seizures, including seizures experienced by people who do not have epilepsy. Some people find that nicotine and/or caffeine use makes their epilepsy worse.

Illegal drugs, particularly cocaine, can cause seizures. They also have a high potential for interacting with prescription medications or interfering with their effects.

The ketogenic diet

This diet plan is a nutritionist's nightmare: it includes almost no starches or sugars. Instead, you consume one gram of protein for every four grams of fat. The body is then forced to burn fat for energy rather than carbohydrates, causing it to produce an abundance of waste products called ketones. These ketones somehow suppress seizure activity in about 30 percent of children with refractory epilepsy and reduce the number of seizures of about half of the remaining number. How this happens is unknown, although it may have to do with an increased number of bicarbonate ions produced in response to high levels of acid in the body (acidosis).[17]

The ketogenic diet is prescribed most frequently for children who have serious seizure disorders, but who are not candidates for surgery. Adults with refractory epilepsy are often curious about whether the ketogenic diet has promise for them. Others may wonder if a modified version of the diet might help improve their seizure control. It is fairly rare for adults to be placed on this diet, although many adults have chosen to incorporate aspects of the diet (higher than normal fat intake, for example) into their eating plans on their own. That's not a wise decision—medical experts say that under no circumstances should this diet be tried without close medical supervision. Not only is the ketogenic diet potentially dangerous to your health in terms of increasing your risk of heart attack and other problems, it's pretty hard to make it appetizing. Each food portion must be carefully weighed, and foods must be given in specific combinations. It is very high in fats, and weight gain may be an unavoidable side effect. Careful supplementation with vitamins is necessary to ensure proper nutrition, and fiber intake must be monitored for digestive health.

Sally, mother of 9-year-old Kay, says the ketogenic diet has been both worthwhile and difficult:

> My daughter is on the keto diet, and we were told by her dietitian that the whole meal needs to be eaten at once. At the beginning that took about an hour to finish. If it's too hard to finish all the prescribed foods at once, talk to your dietitian and ask if your child can be switched to four meals instead of three—but don't change anything without the program's knowledge and support. My daughter's diet has been changed by reducing the ratio twice and increasing the calories and protein once. She has always been a very picky eater, and her keto team told me that they never have had someone so challenging before.

For many of those with intractable seizure disorders, the ketogenic diet is worth the risks. A medical center that specializes in epilepsy treatment should be able to provide guidance and expert nutritional advice if this option is recommended for you or your child. The Johns Hopkins Epilepsy Center (http://hopkins.med.jhu.edu/HealthcarePros/neuro/epilepsy/keto.html) has been at the forefront of research, and it provides information to persons, families, and practitioners.

Persons on the ketogenic diet should not take carnitine (and its precursors lysine and methionine) unless they are directed to do so by a physician, because these amino acids minimize ketone buildup.

Casein-free and gluten-free diets

Quite a few people with neurological problems seem to have problems metabolizing casein (milk protein) and/or gluten (the protein found in wheat and several other grains). In fact, the relationship between this type of metabolic difference and epilepsy has been known since at least the 1920s. For those with either of these digestive problems, eliminating one or both of these proteins from the diet often results in symptom improvements.

Sometimes people with epilepsy have celiac disease, Crohn's disease, or inflammatory bowel disorder (IBD), serious bowel conditions that occur with more frequency in people with neurological problems. Some researchers theorize that since the nervous system and immune system arise from the same fetal tissue, genetic differences or damage that might affect that developing tissue is likely to lead to problems in both areas.

The digestive problems involved with celiac disease and related disorders appear to be autoimmune in nature—the body apparently attacks its own tissue in a misguided attempt to get rid of these foreign proteins. Celiac disease has a particularly close association with disturbances in the parietal and occipital lobes, although the reason for this correlation is not yet known.[18] For people with these conditions, avoiding these substances and treating the inflammation medically usually results in dramatic improvement.

Lisa Lewis has written an excellent book on the topic of casein- and gluten-free diets for children with neurological problems, *Special Diets for Special Kids* (1998, Future Horizons). She also maintains two web sites (*http://members. aol.com/lisas156/index.htm* and *http://www.autismndi.com*). More information about casein-free and gluten-free diets for people of all ages, including recipes, can be found in books written for people with celiac disease. Two other sites of interest, maintained by Don Wiss, are a list of web-based resources for gluten-free diets (*http://www.gluten-free.org*) and the No Milk Page (*http://www. panix.com/~nomilk*). See Appendix A for more information.

Dental care

There's nothing "alternative" about preventing medication-induced damage to your dental heath—if you take medications like Dilantin (phenytoin) or calcium channel blockers, it's simply a must. Don't accept the idea that gaining seizure control with certain AEDs makes gingival hyperplasia (gum overgrowth) inevitable. Recent studies have shown that a special program of intensive dental hygiene can keep your smile looking great.[19]

The gums of people with gingival hyperplasia become enlarged. That creates pockets where bacteria thrive out of reach of your toothbrush, leading to gum disease, bleeding, increased amounts of plaque, cavities, and bone loss. Along with good brushing, more frequent plaque removal by a dental hygienist is helpful, as is using a special mouthwash. Studies have found improvements with a liquid folic acid preparation[20] or with chlorhexidine mouthwash, which actually retards the gum growth itself.[21] Chlorhexidine, available only by prescription, can cause enamel staining.

Consult your dentist about setting up a consistent program of care. He may be able to suggest special brushing techniques or appliances that can protect your teeth and gums.

Hair and skin care

Hair loss and thinning is a significant problem for many people who take AEDs. Vitamin supplements can usually prevent this problem, but you may not be thrilled with how your hair looks in the meantime.

New ingredients in hair-care products can make your hair shinier and thicker-looking, although you should generally avoid drugstore products that use waxes for this purpose. The best place to go for advice is a licensed beautician or barber—both receive extensive training in taking care of hair problems. They can suggest products and hairstyles that minimize thinness and dullness while your hair recovers.

Some people taking AEDs have another hair problem—too much hair growing where it shouldn't (like on a woman's chin, upper lip, or abdomen). Called hirsutism, this can pose a particular dilemma for women taking medications like Dilantin. Hirsutism is a sign that your body is generating too much of the male hormone androgen. It may seem like a cosmetic issue only, but it can be a sign of bigger problems. The same hormonal changes that lead to extra hair growth can also cause polycystic ovary syndrome (PCOS), which can in turn increase your risk for endometrial cancer and reproductive problems. Weight gain and diabetes are also associated with hirsutism. If you notice unusual hair growth on your face or body while taking an AED, ask your doctor to evaluate these on a regular basis.

As for the unwanted hair itself, removal is not difficult. Shaving or drugstore hair-removal formulas such as Neet are fine for excessive body hair, although they can be time-consuming. Waxing is another way to remove unwanted facial hair. A thin layer of wax is spread on a small area of the skin, a piece of cloth is placed on top of the wet wax, and when the wax dries a few seconds later the esthetician pulls it off, taking the hair with it. It stings a lot, especially the first time, but it leaves the skin hair-free for a long period.

Although home waxing kits are available, professionals in the field don't recommend them. For one thing, it's hard to wax yourself. For another, sanitary conditions are important when having this procedure done, and a skin-care professional will also know what to do if hair removal is complicated by other issues, such as skin rashes. If money is a concern, a local beauty school may be able to provide waxing services at very low prices. Otherwise, any licensed esthetician can do the job in a salon or sometimes in your home.

Electrolysis, a procedure that uses electricity to remove hair at the root, is another option, although it can't prevent hair from growing back when that growth is being stimulated by a medication.

Minor skin rashes are fairly common in people using AEDs—anywhere from 7 to 12 percent of persons on some drugs report a particular type of basically harmless but unsightly rash. Called a morbilliform rash, it's a pink, blotchy rash resembling the early stage of measles. It usually appears in people who have just started a medication. The most common cause is a starting dose that's too high, causing an allergy-like reaction. Unless the AED is discontinued, the rash can get worse. Doctors often recommend stopping the medication and using an antihistamine like Benadryl to clear up the outbreak.[22] Medications should never be stopped without your doctor's approval, and antihistamines can actually cause seizures in some people.

Some rashes associated with AEDs are serious, even life-threatening. If you ever experience fever, facial swelling, swollen lymph nodes, blister-like lesions, or peeling skin in connection with a rash, don't wait for a doctor's appointment—go straight to an emergency room. These may be signs of a life-threatening condition caused by medication.

Bringing it all together

As you explore complementary therapies, always keep in mind that "natural" does not mean "harmless." Whenever a vitamin or supplement is powerful enough to heal or prevent illness, it also has the power to harm if misused. Be sure to work closely with your physician or a nutritionist if you are trying anything more complex than taking a daily multivitamin or reducing stress. These professionals can help you avoid mistakes caused by the interaction between complementary therapies and prescription medications.

Also, beware of claims you read in advertisements, in magazine and newspaper articles, or on the Internet. Check the credentials of alternative practitioners before you take their advice, especially if it involves expensive tests or remedies. Be doubly doubtful if a complementary practitioner encourages you to avoid prescription medications. None of the herbal remedies or other alternative treatments available today hold out the promise of a cure for epilepsy. In fact, if you see or hear such claims made, that should immediately make you highly suspicious of the source.

Most importantly, don't let having a seizure disorder become the central fact of your life. Good medical care is crucial for anyone with a chronic health condition, but in the end, living with seizures is all about living, period. Hang onto your sense of humor and your sense of self-worth. Reach out to your family and friends, and let them know when you need help as well as when you're able to handle things on your own. Reach out to others experiencing the same challenges, because they understand where you're coming from and can help you make good choices. It may seem like a cliché, but a positive mental attitude can sometimes do more for your quality of life than the latest medication.

CHAPTER 7

Healthcare and Insurance

HEALTHCARE CAN BE DIFFICULT to get and manage for people who have seizure disorders. This chapter explains how to access the best care through your existing health plan, as well as how to get care if you do not have adequate insurance coverage.

You don't have to have health insurance for this chapter to be useful. It covers private insurance, including health maintenance organizations (HMOs) and other forms of managed care; public health insurance plans; and alternatives to health insurance as well. It also describes typical insurance roadblocks and shows you how to get around them.

Because public assistance in the US and some other countries is closely tied to eligibility for public health benefits, it also covers SSI (Supplemental Security Income) disability income and other benefits that may be available to people whose seizures prevent them from working, and for families with disabled children.

Private insurance: The American way

In the US and other countries where private medical insurance is the norm, the system can be hard to deal with even under the best of circumstances. Each insurance company offers multiple plans with various rates and benefits, and there's no central oversight. As a result, your diagnosis may come with an unpleasant surprise: the healthcare services you need aren't covered, even though you have paid your insurance premiums. Some insurance plans specifically refuse to cover any neurological disorder, and in many cases it's legal for insurers to make that choice.

Some companies try to serve people with partial seizures within mental-health programs, which may or may not be appropriate to their needs, and limit access to neurologists and other specialists. Others may have no qualified "in-plan" practitioners but refuse to make outside referrals, or they may limit plan members to a certain number of outpatient visits or inpatient hospital days each year, regardless of what they actually need. In other cases, your plan may cover all of the medical services you need.

Making insurance choices

Whenever you are in the position of choosing a new insurance plan, try to find out in advance the plan's coverage of treatment for partial seizure disorders. If there is a local epilepsy treatment center, do they accept the plan you're considering? How about the neurologist or psychiatrist you would most like to see?

Although doctors are rarely willing to speak ill of specific insurers, their office staff may not be as circumspect. Ask about whether the firm you're considering cooperates with them at billing time, buries them in unnecessary paperwork, or has a reputation for denying services the doctor requests. You can tell a lot about an insurance company or HMO by how it treats its business partners—and that's what doctors and their staff members are when it comes to healthcare plans.

In the absence of a plan that definitely covers the practitioners and facilities you want, your best bet is one with an out-of-network clause. These plans allow you to choose your own providers if you can't find the right professional on the list of preferred providers or HMO members. You will generally pay more for out-of-plan visits, but you also won't have to run the referral gauntlet as often. The cost of using these providers regularly may be more than your budget will bear, however.

Theresa, mother of 14-year-old Bryce, has chosen this type of plan:

> We've never had an HMO; we've had a plan where we had some choices. I don't really have any restrictions with my plan, so we've always been able to have access to people that we felt comfortable with. That's why I've kept this particular plan—I don't want to always have to justify who Bryce needs to see. We have changed neurologists a couple of times over the years, and that hasn't been a problem.

If your employer does not offer insurance that covers out-of-network providers or other needed services, take up the issue with the human resources or benefits department (or in small companies, the boss). When the cost is spread over a group, expanded benefits may not be very expensive. You can also make a very persuasive case that providing better coverage will keep employees on the job more days, because they will be less likely to need long periods off work due to health problems or caring for a sick family member.

Insurance for families or individuals affected by any long-term disability is very hard to get in the private market (i.e., without going through an employer). It's available, but premium costs can be extraordinarily high. If you are leaving a job that provides you with health insurance for one that does not, pursue a COBRA plan. These allow you to continue your coverage after leaving employment. You will pay the full rate, including the contribution previously made by your employer, but it will still be less than what you'd pay as an individual customer.

Maintaining continuous health insurance coverage is critical to prevent being locked out of healthcare by pre-existing conditions. If a COBRA plan is not available, other lower-cost possibilities include group plans offered by trade associations, unions, clubs, and other organizations. You might also look into public health insurance options, which are discussed later in this chapter.

Managing managed care

In most HMOs and other managed care providers, doctors earn more if their patients stay healthy. In many ways, this makes more sense than rewarding doctors for keeping their patients sick. It removes the financial incentive for ordering unnecessary tests or padding the bill with extra office visits—at least, that's the theory.

For patients with long-term disabilities, however, the reality of managed care is that sometimes you may be perceived as an obstacle in the way of your physician's profits.

There are four basic rules for managing your insurance affairs, whether you're dealing with an HMO, another type of managed-care organization, an old-style "fee for service" arrangement, or a public health agency. Following these steps can help you be more secure when dealing with care providers and insurers:

- Learn how the system works.
- Document everything.
- Form a partnership with your healthcare providers.
- Appeal when necessary.

Learn how the system works

Informed insurance consumers are a rarity. Most people look at the glossy plan brochure and the provider list when their insurance first kicks in, but unless something goes wrong, that's about as much as they want to know. If you suspect that you may need to buck the system, however, you'll need a copy of the firm's master policy.

This document, which specifies everything that is and isn't covered, can be obtained through your employer's human resources office (for employer-provided insurance or COBRA plans administered by a former employer) or from the insurance company's customer relations office (for health insurance that you buy directly from the insurer). Read it. It will be tough going, but the results will be worthwhile.

If you need help interpreting this document, disability advocacy organizations and insurance-related sites on the Web can help. For a list of some helpful organizations, see Appendix A, *Resources*.

Find out in detail what the chain of command is for your healthcare provider and your insurer. You'll need to know exactly who to call and what to do if you need a referral to a specialist, hospitalization, or emergency services.

Document everything

You should keep copies of all your bills, reports, evaluations, test results, and other medical records. You should also keep records of when and how your insurance payments were made. This information will be essential if you have a dispute with your healthcare provider or insurer.

You'll also need to document personal conversations and phone calls. You needn't tape-record these, although if a dispute has already begun this can be a good idea (make sure to let the other party know that you are recording, of course). Simply note the date and time of your call or conversation, whom you spoke with, and what was said or decided. If a service or treatment is promised in a phone conversation, it's a good idea to send a letter or fax documenting the conversation. For example:

> *Dear Dr. Hippocrates:*
>
> *When we spoke on Tuesday, you promised to authorize a referral to Dr. Pauling at the City Hospital Neurology Center for my sleep-deprived EEG and neurological exam. Please fax a copy of the referral form to me*

at xxx-xxxx when it is finished, as well as to Dr. Pauling at xxx-xxxx.
Thanks again for your help.

Referral forms are especially important. Most managed-care firms send a copy to both the patient and the provider. This document usually has a referral number on it. Be sure to bring your referral form when you first see a new provider. If the provider has not received his or her copy of the form, your copy and the referral number can ensure that you'll still be seen and that payment can be processed. Without it, you may be turned away.

Form a partnership with your healthcare providers

Money is a motivator for doctors and other healthcare providers, but most of them also care about helping their patients. Your providers are the most powerful allies you have. Give them additional information about partial seizures if they need it, and make sure they know your case well. Let them know how important their help is. They may not be able to provide direct epilepsy treatment, but they do have the power to write referrals, recommend and approve certain treatments, and advocate on your behalf within the managed-care organization.

Don't rely on your providers completely, however. They have many patients, some of whose needs will likely take precedence over yours. A life-or-death emergency or a large caseload may cause paperwork or meetings on your behalf to be overlooked temporarily or even forgotten.

Another staff member, such as a nurse or office assistant, may be able to keep your provider on track, but you will have to be persistent. Make sure that you return calls, provide accurate information, and keep the provider's needs in mind. For example, if you have information for your doctor about a new medication, summarize it on one page, and attach the relevant studies or journal articles. The doctor can then quickly scan the basics in her office and read the rest when time permits.

Appeal

Would you believe that 70 percent of insurance coverage and claims denials are never appealed? It's true. Most healthcare consumers are so discouraged by the initial denial that they don't pursue it further.

However, all insurance companies and managed-care entities have an internal appeal process, and it's worth your while to be part of the persistent 30 percent. The appeals process should be explained in the master plan. If it's not, call the insurance company's customer service office or your employer's human resources department for information.

A grievance or appeal is not the same thing as a complaint! Companies can ignore complaints at their leisure, as they do not require a legal response. Grievances and appeals do have legal status, and healthcare consumers are entitled to have matters addressed if they are presented in this way. Grievances should be made in writing, and clearly marked "grievance" at the top of the document.

When you file a formal grievance, the managed-care entity will convene a grievance committee made up of people not involved in your problem. This committee will meet to consider the matter, usually within 30 days of receiving your written complaint. Particularly in HMOs, where the committee is usually made up mostly of physicians, your medical arguments may fall upon receptive ears.

It's unlikely that you will be personally present at an insurance company or HMO appeal. You can send written material to support your appeal, such as medical studies that support your position. It's best if your physician or care provider also writes a letter of support, explaining why they support your request for a specific service.

Some companies have more than one level of grievance resolution, so if you are denied at first, check your plan to see if you can appeal the committee's decision to a higher body. You may have the right to appear in person at this higher-level hearing, to bring an outside representative (such as a disability advocate, outside medical expert, or healthcare lawyer), and to question the medical practitioners involved. In other words, if a second-level procedure is available, it will be more like a trial or arbitration hearing than an informal discussion.

If you are still denied, you may be able to pursue the matter with your state's department of health or insurance commission. If your managed-care plan is part of a public insurance program (for example, if you receive Medicaid or state medical benefits but you have been required to join an HMO), you can also appeal through a state agency. If you get your insurance through your employer, your company's benefits manager may be able to help.

Semi-sneaky tips

Some people are better at managing managed care than others. The following suggestions may be a little shady, but they have worked for certain managed-care customers:

- Subvert voicemail and phone queues. If you are continually routed into a voicemail system and your calls are never returned, or if you are left on hold forever, don't passively accept it. Start punching buttons when you are stuck in voicemail or on hold, in hope of reaching a real person. If you get an operator, ask for Administration (the claims and marketing departments never seem to have enough people to answer the phone). Nicely ask the operator to transfer you directly to an appropriate person who can help, not to the department in general. The old "gosh, I just keep getting lost and cut off in your phone system" ploy may do the trick.

- Whenever you speak to someone at your HMO, especially if it's a claims representative, ask for her full name and direct phone number. It will make her feel more accountable for resolving your problem, because she knows you'll call her back directly if she doesn't.

- If you can't get help from a claims or customer service representative, ask for his supervisor. If you're told that he isn't available, get the supervisor's full name, direct phone line, and mailing address. Simply asking for this information sometimes makes missing supervisors magically appear.

- Use humor when you can. It defuses situations that are starting to get ugly and humanizes you to distant healthcare company employees.

- Explain why your request is urgent, and do so in terms that non-doctors can understand. For example, if receiving a certain treatment now could mean avoiding expensive hospitalization later, that's an argument that even junior assistant accountants can comprehend.

- Whatever you do, stay calm. If you yell at managed-care people, they'll be angry instead of sympathetic. That doesn't mean being unemotional. Sometimes you can successfully make a personal appeal. You can act confused instead of angry when you are denied assistance for no good reason. You may also want to make it clear that you're gathering information in a way that indicates legal action—for instance, asking how to spell names and asking where official documents should be sent.

Some plans have a special-needs liaison, an employee whose job is making sure that members with disabilities are cared for properly. Most special-needs liaisons act more like a resource person than an ombudsman, but the best of them can help you strategize to get what you need.

Melissa, mother of 10-year-old Chris, explains how her insurance company's liaison helped:

> *Chris is on a public insurance plan, based on a Medicaid waiver that gives us a choice of five HMOs. We were having real problems getting to see a child neurologist. I called the special-needs coordinator, and she walked me through the process of how to get a referral and made sure we didn't have to wait any longer than we already had. She also made some phone calls on our behalf. I'm not great at dealing with bureaucracy, so her help was really appreciated.*

Fighting denial of care

Refusal of appropriate care is the top insurance complaint among people coping with any form of disability. You can fight denial of care, but it isn't easy. Begin by asking the insurance company's claims department for a written copy of the denial of coverage or services. Make sure that the reason you were given verbally is also the reason given in this document.

Your next stop is the insurance company's own documents. Somewhere in the fine print of the master policy that you should already have in your files, you will probably find a provision stating that if any of the company's policies are unenforceable based on state law, they cannot be asserted. Most insurance company claims adjusters know very little about state insurance law. Your job is to educate yourself and then educate them.

Now you need to find out what your state says about coverage in general and about epilepsy (or mental illness, if you have a dual diagnosis or have been shunted off into the mental health system) in particular. The answer may be found in actual legislation. Epilepsy is not normally included in the list of conditions covered under the mental health parity laws now found in some states, but the rationale behind those laws is that any brain illness deserves equal treatment. Laws protecting the disabled against discrimination may also have bearing.

Your state's insurance commission—every state has its own, and there's no federal insurance commission—will also have policies about coverage. Remember, actual state law trumps state policy statements every time. State laws may be more restrictive than federal regulations, in which case the state prevails. If state laws are less restrictive than federal mandates, the federal government prevails. Insurance commission staff members should also be able to help you with general questions about what your state requires coverage for, and they can tell you about any protections that may be written into state insurance, healthcare, or consumer protection laws.

Your state's Epilepsy Foundation chapter will probably already have the information you need on hand, call the national office, listed in Appendix A, if you need contact information. If not, you'll have to start researching on your own. If you have Internet access, you may find state laws, some public policies, and possibly insurance commission decisions online. You could also call your state representative's office and ask a staff member to research this issue for you.

If you can show your insurance company that it is trying to assert a provision that violates a state or federal law, it should back down and provide treatment. Legal arguments of the sort needed to secure coverage can be hard for a layperson to craft. Advocacy groups may be able to help you write a persuasive letter of appeal on legal grounds. Some people have convinced their state representative or a member of Congress to intervene on their behalf, especially if the problem involves a public insurance program or facility.

Formal arbitration is another possibility, although experienced advocates warn that, since arbitrators are paid by the healthcare plans, it's a tough arena for consumers. In most cases, you can't recover your legal costs in arbitration, although they can reach $50,000 or more. Most consumer-law cases in the courts are taken by lawyers who work on contingency, meaning that you don't pay unless you win a financial settlement, so it's hard to secure legal help for arbitration. Arbitration can actually cost consumers more than a court trial, and if it is binding arbitration, it may prevent you from pursuing help through the court system if the decision goes against you.[1]

Taking your insurance company to court is something that you should consider only as a last resort. It's expensive, and it takes so long for a decision to come down and then be implemented that your current healthcare crisis may have passed long before the gavel bangs. If you have the means and the gumption, don't be dissuaded from making things better for others. Just don't pin all your hopes on a quick resolution by a judge.

In some cases your state disability protection and advocacy group (see the listing for the National Association of Protection and Advocacy Systems in Appendix A) can provide legal advice or even representation, and there are lawyers willing to take insurance cases on contingency.

Your best bet is to research the reason your insurance company or provider is denying care and find persuasive evidence that can change the decisions made by its staff.

Denial for plan limits

If your insurance company only provides treatment for partial seizure disorders as part of a limited mental health or nervous disorders benefit, you can challenge that limitation. Epilepsy is biologically based and should be treated the same as diabetes, heart trouble, or any other medical condition.

Your neurologist or psychiatrist can help plead your case by providing hard evidence of your condition, such as EEG results, CAT scans, and test results. Your doctor can also explain how much more cost-effective consistent treatment for your seizures is—particularly by showing the insurance company what the financial risk is of going without the treatment. Hospitalization, for example, is far more expensive than adequate medication and case management.

Getting coverage for new treatments

Almost all insurance plans bar coverage for experimental treatments. Some do have a "compassionate care" exception, which comes into play when regular treatments have been tried unsuccessfully and the plan's medical advisors agree that the experimental treatment might work. This exception is sometimes made available to people with refractory epilepsy.

Cheri, age 29, had to appeal to her insurance company to get the cost for her vagus nerve stimulator covered:

> My insurance company is considered by many to be one of the best in the country. However, when I went to them for coverage on the vagus nerve stimulator implant, they did all they could to avoid it. When they realized that "pre-existing condition" didn't apply in my case, they

decided that the VNS was still experimental in their book and not cov-
ered. I was with several neurologists for this procedure, one of whom in
particular had fought this battle a few times before. It took a while, but
the appeal came out successfully. In the end, I paid only a few hundred
dollars instead of $35,000.

So what do you do to pay for promising new treatments, such as newly developed medications that aren't on your insurance company's approved list? You either pay out-of-pocket, or you work closely with your physician to get around the experimental treatment exclusion.

Your physician may have to prepare a "letter of medical necessity" to support your request—or this task may fall to you. This letter must include:

- The diagnosis for which the service, equipment, or medication is needed.

- The specific symptom or function that the service, equipment, or medication will treat.

- A full description of the service, equipment, or medication and how it will help the patient.

- If the service, equipment, or medication is new or experimental, evidence (medical studies, journal articles, etc.) to support your request.

- If there are less expensive or traditionally used alternatives to the new or experimental service, equipment, or medication, well-supported reasons that these alternatives are not appropriate for you.

Public healthcare in the US

Some people in the US have an extremely serious health insurance problem: they just can't get any. If this ever-growing group includes you, the main publicly funded option is Medicaid, with or without a waiver program. The federal government also has the TRICARE plan for those in current military service and their dependents and, through the Veterans Administration, coverage for former military personnel.

Medicaid and Medicare

Medicaid is the federal health insurance program for eligible individuals who are not senior citizens. It will pay for doctor and hospital bills, including consultations with neurologists and psychiatrists; six prescription medications per month; physical, occupational, and speech therapy; and adaptive equipment. You can get Medicaid by becoming eligible for SSI (see the next section) or, in some cases, by qualifying for state health plans that are based on Medicaid.

Medicaid is one of the few insurance plans that will pay for in-home therapy services, therapeutic foster care, partial hospitalization or day treatment, crisis services, and long-term hospitalization or residential care for people with disabilities. Although it is excessively bureaucratic, it is in many ways superior to private insurance coverage for people who have disabilities. .

Medicare is a health insurance program for senior citizens. If you are receiving Social Security benefits due to your age, you should also be receiving Medicare.

SSI and SSDI

Supplemental Security Income (SSI) is a benefit program available to severely disabled children of low-income families. In all states, Washington DC, and the Northern Marianas Islands, disabled adults and children who qualify for SSI also qualify for healthcare coverage through the federal Medicaid plan.

Adult benefits are currently about $530 per month; children and adults living in another person's household receive less. This money is only to be used for the direct needs of the disabled individual; it is not family income per se. You will need to keep receipts for all your expenditures. Some states supplement SSI.

Another program, Social Security Disability Income (SSDI), is available to adults who have worked and paid into the Social Security system, but who have since become disabled and can demonstrate an inability to work. If married, the disabled adult and spouse must meet the stringent income and asset limits. In some states and Washington, DC, SSI or SSDI can make you eligible for Medicaid.

There are specific medical requirements for SSI or SSDI eligibility for people with epilepsy. At this time, the regulations require that, despite complying with medical treatment for three months or more, you continue to have one tonic-clonic seizure per month and/or one seizure involving alteration or loss of consciousness per week.

To apply for SSI, SSDI, and/or Medicaid, go to your nearest Social Security office or call the Social Security hotline at (800) 772-1213 for an eligibility pre-screening. If you are given a green light by the eligibility screener, your next step is making an initial interview appointment and filling out a long form. This form asks dozens of difficult questions, including information about every physician or clinic that might have your medical records or test results, and information about your previous contacts with public health agencies. It helps to provide copies of as many of your health records as you can.

If you need help in completing this form (and many people do), a social worker or someone from a disability advocacy group may be able to assist you.

Make sure your forms and records are complete when your initial interview takes place. You can be interviewed in person or over the phone. Most experienced applicants say in-person interviews are best, but they aren't always possible. If you choose a phone interview, it is very important to keep careful records and have phone numbers and addresses for your doctors and (for parents) school personnel handy.

During the interview, the Social Security representative will go over the disability report with you. She may ask additional questions. Some of them may seem rather prying to people who have never applied for any type of government assistance. In fact, the application process has become increasingly adversarial over the past two decades. You may get the distinct impression that the person interviewing you thinks you are trying to con them—and your impression may be right.

If the Social Security caseworker is unsure about whether you are disabled enough for SSI or SSDI eligibility, she may order an Individualized Functional Assessment (IFA). This is a review of your medical documentation by a state agency or Social Security representatives, sometimes accompanied by interviews and observation by doctors working for the state or at the direction of Social Security.

Most applicants for SSI and SSDI are rejected on their first try. You do have the right to appeal this denial, however—and you should, because a high percentage of appeals succeed. In addition, successful appellants get a lump sum equal to the payments they should have received, had their original application been properly approved. You must appeal within 60 days of denial.

If your application is denied, contact a disability advocacy agency through the National Association of Protection and Advocacy Systems, which is listed in Appendix A. These publicly funded agencies can help you through the application process, and most can provide legal assistance if you need to appeal. You can also use a lawyer, who will be paid part of any award.

Additional information about the SSI program for children with disabilities is available online at *http://www.ssas.com*, the site of the Social Security Advisory Service.

Medicaid waivers

The reason someone would need a Medicaid waiver is that SSI is usually an income-dependent program. A waiver sets aside the income limits. If you or your spouse earns more than the regulations allow, a disabled spouse or child will not be eligible for SSI. In some cases, family income will reduce the amount of SSI received to as low as one dollar per month, but the beneficiary will get full medical coverage. Others must apply for a special income-limit waiver—those for disabled children are colloquially known as Katie Beckett waivers, named after a severely disabled child whose parents' pleas inspired the program.

The Katie Beckett waiver program is part of a larger category of Medicaid waiver permissions for the states under the general title of Home and Community-Based Services, or 1915(c), waivers. These waiver programs are administered at a state level. Some states have severely limited the number of waivers they will allow; some have created their own disability-specific waiver pools for conditions like cerebral palsy and autism, and a few do not offer any waivers at all. Contact your county's Child and Family Services (CFS) department and ask for an appointment with a Medicaid worker, who can help you learn about and apply for waiver programs that may be available in your state.

The appointment to apply for a waiver will be long, and the questions will be intrusive, so be prepared. You will need copious documentation, including the following:

- In most states, a rejection letter from SSI citing your income as the reason for rejection.

- Your or your child's birth certificate and Social Security number.

- Proof of income (check stubs or a CFS form filled out and signed by your and/or your spouse's employer, and possibly income tax forms).

- Names, addresses, and phone numbers of all physicians who have examined you or your child.

- Bank account and safety deposit box numbers, and amounts in these accounts.

- List of other assets and their value, including your house and car.

- A DMA6 medical report and a physician referral form signed by the doctor who knows you or your child best (CFS will provide these forms).

If you have a caseworker with your county's mental health offices, or if you regularly work with someone at a regional center or in an early intervention program, this person may be able to help you navigate the SSI, Medicaid, and waiver process. State-by-state information about waiver programs is available online at *http://www.hcfa.gov/medicaid/hpg4.htm*.

If you have specific problems with accessing appropriate medical benefits under Medicaid, state health plans, or other public healthcare plans, your caseworker or an advocate from the Epilepsy Foundation may be able to help. If your problems are of a legal nature, such as outright refusal of services or discrimination, call your state Bar Association and ask for its pro bono (free) legal help referral service, or contact the National Association of Protection and Advocacy Systems (see Appendix A). This national organization can put you in touch with your state's protection and advocacy agency, which provides free advice and legal help for issues related to disability. You can also consult the Health Law Project at (800) 274-3258.

State and local public health plans

All 50 US states, Puerto Rico, Guam, and several US holdings participate in the federal program known as State Children's Insurance Plans (SCHIP, also known as Title XXI), which offers uninsured children the same or similar benefits as Medicaid does. Each state's plan is slightly different, and some may not be fully operational as of this writing (summer 2000). Several states also have income-based state plans for adults on public assistance or in low-wage occupations, and some offer insurance "pools" for people who have been refused coverage due to preexisting conditions. Most of these state plans make innovative use of federal Medicaid monies, combined with state funding. For updated information about some state programs, see the national SCHIP web site at *http://www.hcfa.gov/init/children.htm*. You can also call your state health department.

In some areas, city or county health programs are available, either in the form of insurance or simply access to a network of public clinics that operate on a sliding-scale fee basis.

TRICARE

TRICARE Standard is the health insurance program provided to active duty and retired members of the US military under the age of 65 and their families. A special service within TRICARE, the Program for Persons with Disabilities, can help you with special medical needs, including care for a family member with a disability or developmental delay. TRICARE also includes dental benefits and access to Department of Defense pharmacies. A second program called TRICARE Extra offers more benefits.

Retired service members over age 65 may move into a special Medicare program (TRICARE Prime) operated by the Department of Defense, although this area of benefits is changing.

The problem with public health plans

Coverage is a fine thing, but what happens when no one will accept you as a patient? This is the situation faced by millions of Americans who have government-provided healthcare. You may find yourself limited to using county health clinics or public hospitals, and to those private providers who are willing to work for cut-rate fees. Medicaid and its cousins pay healthcare providers less than private insurers do, and there's no law that says a given provider must take patients with public insurance. The latest wrinkle in some states is that even public health clinics are refusing the uninsured unless it's an emergency situation.

Pat says a referral to a neurologist was very hard to get when she used the Oregon Health Plan (OHP), a Medicaid-based public health insurance program:

> When I first went to an OHP doctor, I hadn't had an EEG in several years. I expected that, since I had epilepsy, the doctor would want me to see a neurologist and have an EEG—sort of a check-up. But the doctor said, as best as I can recall, that she couldn't refer me unless I was having "breakthrough seizures," because seeing a neuro would be very costly to OHP. Soon after that, she changed my medication from Dilantin to Depakote, but I don't know why, since I was having no discernible problems with the Dilantin. Even my pharmacist later told me that he was surprised.

Soon after she changed my medication, I did have seizures. However, even though I was having seizures, she still wouldn't let me see a neurologist. She just switched me back to Dilantin...Perhaps if I had ranted and raved some, I might've gotten my way, but needless to say, I didn't go back to her. I started seeing another doctor, who I liked a lot, and the first time I asked to see a neuro, he gave me the referral.

Perhaps the first doctor wanted to keep costs down so OHP would give her a Cheapness in Medicine Prize. Perhaps OHP had complained that she'd been referring too many people to specialists. Or maybe the second doctor thought I should see a neuro, especially since I'd had the seizures and hadn't been to one in a while.

Some public facilities are run-down, understaffed, and hectic as a result of high demand and low budgets. In fact, the emergency rooms of some public hospitals are downright frightening on weekend nights! Familiarize yourself with all of the options covered by your public healthcare plan. You may have more choices than you originally thought. In some cases you may have the option to join one or more HMO plans, receiving the same benefits as non-subsidized HMO members. Check with other recipients or local advocacy groups if you are offered this choice—some of these plans do a good job of caring for disabled clients, while others are not preferable to plain old Medicaid or state healthcare.

Sadly, there is also an anti-welfare attitude abroad amongst some healthcare workers, who may not know or care what financial and medical troubles drove you to need public healthcare or income help. You shouldn't have to tolerate substandard or unbusinesslike treatment from providers. If it happens and you can't work things out with the provider directly, ask your caseworker about complaint options.

Other public assistance for the disabled

While Canada, all western European nations, and many other countries provide family support allowances to encourage one parent to stay home with young children, the US government has cut support even to single parents, and it provides extraordinarily low allowances when they are available. This policy affects the parents of children with disabilities particularly harshly.

Between the 1950s and the 1980s, single, low-income parents of children with disabilities tended to receive Aid to Families with Dependent Children (AFDC, welfare) and SSI. When put together, income from these two programs permitted them to eke out a living. While they remained well below the poverty line, they could generally obtain housing and adequate food. For many of these families, the most important benefit of receiving public assistance was access to Medicaid.

Welfare reform has changed this picture drastically. The Temporary Assistance for Needy Families (TANF) program, a system of short-term emergency supports, has replaced AFDC. All states have now imposed stringent rules, such as limiting assistance to once in a lifetime, requiring that parents work for their grants, or forcing parents into job-training schemes geared toward a rapid transition to low-wage employment. Although most states have also added childcare services to their offerings to help parents receiving TANF grants transition to the workplace, affordable childcare slots for children and teens with disabilities are almost nonexistent. This leaves even the most determined low-income parent at a severe disadvantage.

Federal law permits exceptions to TANF regulations to be made for some— but not all—parents caring for disabled children, and for parents who are themselves disabled. However, caseworkers are responsible for holding down the number of exemptions to 20 percent or less of their clients, even though as many as a third of families on welfare include either a mother or a child with a serious disability. For more information about this issue, see "Recent Studies of AFDC Recipients Estimate Need for Specialized Child Care" at http://www.welfare-policy.org/childdis.htm.

If you have epilepsy and are parenting, TANF may work for you or against you. Some parents who have let their caseworker know about a health problem that could conceivably affect their ability to care for their children have been exempted from certain regulations or even offered extra help. Others have lost their children to the state. You should see a welfare rights organization or sympathetic social worker before making the decision to tell. They can help you ensure your children's security by approaching the issue knowledgeably.

You can apply for TANF at your county's child and family services department. The program is primarily for single parents, but two-parent families are eligible in some areas and under some circumstances. The amount of the monthly grant varies. It is determined by the county government, which administers TANF programs at the local level. Grants range from around $150 per month in some rural southern counties to about $650 per month in expensive cities like San Francisco, where a small supplemental housing benefit is factored into the grant.

If you are parenting a child whose seizures are severely debilitating, you'll need to provide very complete documentation to get and retain benefits on the basis of needing to provide full-time home care. You can expect to have an eligibility review at least every three months, during which all of your documents will be reviewed and you will be re-interviewed. Generally speaking, you cannot have savings or possessions worth over $1,000, although you may own a modest home and car. You may need to sell a late-model car and other valuables before you can receive benefits. Your grant may be reduced by the amount of other financial assistance you receive. If you find part-time work, your grant may also be reduced by this amount or a portion thereof—some states do have work incentive programs, however. Court-ordered child-support payments to TANF recipients are paid to the county rather than directly to the parent, to offset the cost of the grant.

You may be eligible for food stamps, commodities (free food), and other benefits, such as job training, if you receive TANF. People leaving TANF programs may be eligible for certain short-term benefits, such as subsidized childcare and continued health insurance.

If you need help obtaining public assistance, contact a local welfare rights organization or advocacy group, or contact the National Welfare Monitoring and Advocacy Partnership (NWMAP) for national information and referrals (see Appendix A).

Indirect financial help

In the US, tax deductions have replaced direct financial assistance to the poor in many cases. These benefits are provided once a year, but families coping with the high cost of caring for a disabled child should take advantage of them.

One of the most important tax benefits is the ability to itemize medical deductions on your federal income tax. You can write off not only the direct cost of doctor's visits not covered by health insurance, but also health insurance co-pays and deductibles, out-of-pocket expenses for medications, travel costs related to medical care, and at least some expenses related to attending medical or disability conferences and classes. Self-employed people can deduct most of their health-insurance premiums, even if they don't itemize.

Because itemized deductions limit your federal tax liability, they also reduce your state income taxes, if any (state taxes are usually based on taxable income figures taken from your federal form). Some states have additional tax benefits for the disabled. In Oregon, for example, each disabled child counts as two dependents.

Another important federal tax benefit is the Earned Income Credit (EIC) program. This benefit for the working poor can actually supplement your earnings with a tax rebate, not just a deduction. You can file for EIC on your federal 1040 tax form.

Mortgage interest is also tax-deductible, as most people are aware. Since your home is usually not considered as an asset when determining eligibility for direct financial assistance, such as SSI, this makes home ownership particularly attractive to families coping with disability. Some banks and credit unions have special mortgage programs for low- and moderate-income families. Given the strong financial benefits of home ownership, including the opportunity to keep your housing costs from going up in the future, purchasing a house is very advisable.

Very low income families, including young adults with seizure disorders who rely on SSI or fixed-income trusts, may be able to get additional help in reaching the goal of home ownership from organizations like Habitat for Humanity (see Appendix A). Disability advocacy and social service organizations have recently begun to push to increase the level of home ownership among disabled adults. In some cases the home can be part of a special trust that provides professional management services.

Benefits in Canada

In Canada, the Canada Health Act ensures coverage for all Canadian citizens and for non-citizens who need emergency care. Healthcare regulations are the same nationwide, although providers can be hard to find in the less-populated northern provinces.

To initiate an evaluation for a seizure disorder, see your primary care physician, who can then make a referral to an appropriate specialist. A wide variety of specialists are available through the Canadian health plan, Medicare, which is administered by Health Canada/Santé Canada. Most of the best epileptologists in Canada are affiliated with university hospitals. Waiting lists are a reality, but parents report that calls and letters (especially if they come from the pediatrician or family doctor) can often open doors.

If no qualified providers are available nearby, public assistance programs are available to help patients get expert care elsewhere. This help may include covering transportation costs, housing the patient during evaluation and treatment, and providing regular consultations later on with a doctor closer to home. In practice, however, people in rural Canada sometimes have great difficulty in obtaining adequate care for disabilities.

Patients in Canada also report that privatization and other changes are starting to limit their access to healthcare. Some families are now carrying private insurance to ensure timely and frequent access to care providers.

Canadians in border areas may wish to consult with specialists in the US. Except for rare and pre-approved cases, Medicare will not cover these visits.

Income support is available in Canada for people with disabilities, single parents, and unemployed adults with or without children. The amount of the monthly payment is set at the provincial level. The disability payment varies from a low of about $580 per month in poor provinces like New Brunswick to around $800 per month in more expensive Ontario and British Columbia. Under the Canadian system, payments to parents caring for children, single or otherwise, are higher than those for disabled adults.

To apply for welfare benefits, visit your nearest ministry or department of social services. For disability benefits, regulations vary by province. Typically, you must be 18 years of age or older and have confirmation from a medical practitioner that the impairment exists and will likely continue for at least two years or longer, or that it is likely to continue for at least one year and then reoccur. In addition you must require, as a direct result of a severe mental or physical impairment, one of the following:

- Extensive assistance or supervision in order to perform daily living tasks within a reasonable time

- Unusual and continuous monthly expenditures for transportation, special diets, or other unusual but essential and continuous needs

There are limits on the amount and kinds of savings and other property that a person or family receiving benefits can have.

As in the US, welfare reform is a growing trend in Canada. Some provinces have introduced mandatory workfare programs for single adults and for some parents on welfare. These provisions generally do not apply to people receiving disability benefits, and parents caring for disabled children can usually have welfare-to-work requirements waived or deferred.

Canadians who are denied benefits or who have other problems with the benefits agency can appeal its decisions to an independent tribunal. Some assistance for people with disabilities may also be available at the federal level or from First Nations (Native Canadian) agencies.

Other direct and indirect income assistance is available to Canadians, including income tax benefits. College students with permanent disabilities can have their student loans forgiven and are also eligible for special grants to pay for hiring a note-taker, paying for transportation, and other education-related expenses.

Benefits in the UK

The National Health system in Britain and Scotland has undergone tremendous upheaval over the past three decades. All services were once free to UK citizens, while private-pay physicians were strictly for the wealthy. Public services have since been sharply curtailed, and co-pays have been introduced. Nevertheless, services for people with epilepsy are much better now than they were in the past.

Specialists are accessed through your general practitioner (GP). Referrals to specialists are notoriously difficult to obtain, even for private-pay patients.

In the UK, people with disabilities have access to three major types of direct state benefits. You can apply for these programs at your local Benefits Agency Office:

- The Disability Living Allowance (DLA) is for adults or children with a disability. Parents or carers can apply on behalf of a child. Payment ranges from fifteen to thirty-five pounds per week. The DLA forms are relatively complex, so find an experienced disability advocate to help you fill them out if possible. Your local council may also have staff members who can help you apply.

- Parents and others caring for a child who receives DLA can apply for the Attendants Allowance (also called the Carers Allowance) program as well.

- Any person over five years old who receives DLA can also get a Mobility Allowance, a small sum of money to help them get to medical appointments and meet general transportation needs.

Your local council may also have its own benefits scheme. These may be direct payments, such as a supplemental housing benefit, or tax offsets.

A number of supported work schemes are available for people with disabilities and adults receiving other forms of public assistance. In some cases, these programs are mandatory. If you are parenting a child with a seizure disorder, he should start learning about these programs before school-leaving age.

Teens and young adults attending college or trade school may find themselves in a Catch-22 situation: on some occasions, benefits officers have decided that if they are well enough to go to college, they're well enough to work, and canceled their benefits. You can appeal these and other unfavorable decisions to a Social Security Appeals Tribunal.

Help with disability benefit issues is available from UK groups listed in Appendix A.

Benefits in the Republic of Ireland

Disability Allowance and Disability Benefit are available in Ireland, but they are far from generous. The Department of Social Welfare administers both of them. Disabled students can continue to receive these benefits while attending third-level courses, although they may lose other types of public assistance, such as rent allowance. Maintenance grant (a general benefit for poor families) is not affected by these benefits.

Supported work schemes are available, although your earnings may make you lose your disability benefits. The exception is work that the local welfare officer agrees is "rehabilitative" in nature. Some direct healthcare is available from public or charitable hospitals and clinics in Ireland at low or no cost. In Northern Ireland, there are a number of scholarship and grant programs available to assist students with disabilities. An online report at *http://www.ahead.ie/grants/grants.html#toc* offers more information.

Benefits in Australia

Medicare, the Australian health plan, pays 85 percent of all doctor's fees. It also qualifies Australian citizens for treatment in any public hospital at no cost. Many general practitioners and pediatricians bulk bill: they charge the government directly for all of their patient visits and let the 15 percent co-payment slide. Specialists usually won't bulk bill. Once a certain cost level has been reached, Medicare pays 100 percent of the bill.

Patients can see the physician of their choice without getting a preliminary referral, but many specialists have long waiting lists. Access to qualified practitioners is especially difficult in rural areas, although the emergency healthcare system for rural Australia is enviable. In some situations, patients may be able to access professionals for advice or "virtual consultations" over the Internet, telephone, or even radio.

Medicaid does not cover some prescription medications, and there is a sliding-scale co-payment for those that are.

A variety of income support programs are available to Australian citizens, including direct financial assistance for adults with disabilities, parents caring for children with disabilities, single parents, unemployed single adults, youth, and students. Programs related specifically to disabled citizens and their families include Disability Support Pension, Related Wife Pension, Sickness Allowance, Mobility Allowance, Carer Payment, and Child Disability Allowance.

Employment programs for Australians with disabilities are many and varied, including the Supported Wage System (SWS), which brings the earnings of disabled workers in sheltered workshops or other types of supported or low-wage employment closer to the livability range.

Indirect benefits may also be available under the Disability Services Act in the areas of education, work, recreation, and more.

You can find online information about all of Australia's benefit plans at the Centrelink web site (*http://www.centrelink.gov.au*). To apply for benefits or disability services, contact your local Department of Family and Community Services.

You can get help with disability income and health benefit issues from the support and advocacy organizations listed in Appendix A.

Benefits in New Zealand

About 75 percent of all healthcare in New Zealand is publicly funded. Care is delivered through private physicians who accept payment from the public health system. Treatment at public hospitals is fully covered for all New Zealand citizens and also for Australian and UK citizens living and working in New Zealand. Privatization is a growing trend in New Zealand. Public hospitals and their allied clinics have been recreated as public-private corporations. However, the government still provides most of the funding and regulations for healthcare.

Healthcare and disability services are both provided through a central health authority, which has been making special efforts to improve delivery for the past few years. To start an assessment, patients should first talk to their pediatrician or family physician about a specialist referral. Self-referral is also possible.

Urban patients may have access to group practices centered around Crown (public) hospitals, which often have excellent specialists. Māori patients may access healthcare and assessments through medical clinics centered around traditional iwi (tribal) structures if they prefer.

About 40 percent of the population in New Zealand carries private insurance, primarily for hospitalization or long-term geriatric care only. This insurance is helpful when you need elective surgery and want to avoid waiting lists at public hospitals. It is not needed to access psychiatric care or other direct health or disability services.

New Zealanders complain that waiting lists for assessments and major medical treatments can be excessive. Until recently, patients on waiting lists were not given a firm date for their visits and were expected to be available immediately should an opening occur. A new booking system was recently instituted that is said to be more reliable.

For patients in need of temporary or permanent residential care, volunteer organizations (particularly churches) are heavily involved in running long-term care facilities in New Zealand. These facilities are usually free of charge to the patient or family, although some are reimbursed by public health.

Direct benefits in New Zealand are similar to those provided in Australia, although the payments have historically been much lower. Domestic Purposes Benefit is for single parents, including those with disabled children.

There are also a number of additional services available to the disabled and their carers, including training schemes, supported employment, and recreational assistance. The social safety net in New Zealand is currently being revamped, but services for people with disabilities are expected to expand.

To apply for benefits or services, contact your local Ministry of Social Welfare office, which runs the Income Support program. If you need help with paperwork or appeals, Beneficiary Advisory Services (*http://canterbury.cyberplace. org.nz/community/bas.html*) in Christchurch provides assistance and advocacy, as do a number of disability advocacy groups, particularly the information clearinghouse Disability Information Service (*http://canterbury.cyberplace.co.nz/ community/dis.html*).

Alternatives to insurance

No matter where you live, there are alternatives to expensive medical care. Those who don't have insurance, or whose insurance is inadequate, will want to investigate these resources.

In some cases, creative private-pay arrangements may be possible with psychiatrists and other providers. Parents have traded services or products for care, and others have arranged payment plans or reduced fees based on financial need. The larger the provider, the more likely it is to have a system in place for providing income-based fees. The smaller the provider, the more receptive an individual might be to informal arrangements, including barter.

Hospitals and major clinics usually have social workers on staff who can help you make financial arrangements.

Sources of free or low-cost healthcare or therapeutic services may include:

- Public health clinics, including school-based health clinics
- Public hospitals
- Medical schools and associated teaching hospitals and clinics
- Hospitals and clinics run by religious or charitable orders, such as Lutheran Family Services clinics
- Charitable institutions associated with religious denominations, such as Catholic Charities, the Jewish Aid Society, and the Salvation Army
- United Way, an umbrella fundraising organization for many programs that can often provide referrals

- Children's Home Society, the Boys and Girls Aid Society, and similar local children's aid associations

- Grant programs, both public and private

Medical savings accounts

This is a new healthcare payment option in the US that may have benefits for some children and adults with seizure disorders. A medical savings account (MSA) allows families to put away a certain amount of money specifically for healthcare costs. This income will then be exempted from federal (and in some cases state) income taxes. Unused funds continue to gain tax-free interest. These accounts can be used to pay for insurance deductibles, co-payments, prescriptions, and medical services not covered by insurance.

Families faced with paying out-of-pocket for an expensive residential program or experimental medication might be able to use an MSA to reduce their costs by an impressive percentage. You'll need to check the regulations of the specific MSA plan to see what expenses will qualify.

MSAs are currently available through a wide variety of investment firms, as well as some banks. They are governed by rules similar to those for an Individual Retirement Account (IRA), except that you can make withdrawals as needed for qualified medical expenses. There are limits to how much you can place in an MSA, what expenses it can be withdrawn for, and who can have an MSA. Talk to a financial advisor at your bank or an investment firm for more information about MSAs.

Help with medications

Low-income patients may be able to get their medications for free by providing documentation to charitable programs run by pharmaceutical companies. In the US, the Pharmaceutical Research and Manufacturers of America (PhRMA) publishes a directory of medication assistance programs at *http:// www.phrma.org/patients/*. Alternatively, you or your doctor can call the company that makes your medication to find out about its indigent patient program. Individual company programs are listed in Appendix A.

Most require that you have no insurance coverage for outpatient prescription drugs, that purchasing the medication at its retail price would be a hardship for you due to your income and/or expenses, and that you do not qualify for a government or third-party program that can pay for the prescription. An organization called The Medicine Program at (573) 996-7300 and *http://www.themedicineprogram.com* can help you apply to indigent patient programs.

Doctor's samples

Another source for free medications is your physician's sample cabinet. All you have to do is ask, and hope that the pharmaceutical rep has paid a recent visit. Samples can help tide you over rough financial patches, but you can't rely on getting them monthly.

Mail-order medications

In some cases, you can reduce the cost of your monthly medication bill by using a mail-order or online pharmacy. These pharmacies can fill your prescription and mail it to you, sometimes at a substantial savings. Medications may be available via mail-order within your country or from overseas. The latter option can be surprisingly inexpensive and may provide you with access to medications that normally would not be available where you live.

Your doctor may have to fill out some paperwork before you can use these mail-order services. As with any other transaction by mail or over the Internet, you should check out the company's reputation and quality of service before sending money or using your credit card.

These firms can usually send you a three-month supply in each order. If you are doing business with an overseas pharmacy, check Customs regulations that might prohibit you from importing medication before ordering, especially if the drug is not approved for use in your country.

Some mail-order and online pharmacies were initially created to serve the market for AIDS medications but have since expanded to cover a wide selection. Many will accept health insurance if you have a drug benefit—some will actually cover your medication co-payment as part of the deal.

If you have US military health benefits, contact your TRICARE representative about mail-order arrangements. The main TRICARE-approved mail-order service is Merck-Medco at (800) 903-4680 and *http://www.merck-medco.com/medco/index.jsp*.

Appendix A lists mail-order pharmacies that some patients have worked with successfully.

Clinical trials

Some patients have received excellent medical care by taking part in clinical trials of new medications or treatments. Others have suffered unpleasant side effects or felt that they were treated like guinea pigs. Before enrolling in a clinical trial, make sure that you feel comfortable with the procedure or medication being tested, the professionals conducting the study, and the facility where it will take place. An international listing service for current clinical trials is available at *http://www.centerwatch.com*. You can reach Center-Watch by phone at (617) 247-2327.

Miscellaneous discounts

There are a number of programs around the world that help disabled people get access to computers and the Internet. A list of organizations and programs that provide free or low-cost computers, or free computer help, can be found online at *http://www.dmoz.org/computers/organizations/non-profit/*.

If you or your child needs medical care in a location far from home but you can't afford the cost of a flight or hotel, Appendix A lists resources in the US and Canada that may be able to help.

Similar corporate programs may be available in Europe, Australia, and New Zealand; contact the public relations office of your national airline to find out more. You may also be eligible for an emergency travel grant from a social services agency to cover these needs.

Life and auto insurance

Epilepsy does carry with it a risk of early death from seizure-related accidents, status epilepticus, or the rare and unexplained occurrence known as Sudden Death in Epilepsy (SUDEP). However, this risk is less than 2 percent for all people with epilepsy and far lower for those who experience partial or complex partial seizures only. This is considerably lower than the risks associated with smoking, overuse of alcohol, or even eating a high-fat diet, and yet epilepsy can prevent you from qualifying for some life insurance plans.

If you are buying life insurance on the private market, you'll probably need to hunt around. Some plans may be willing to take you, but only at a higher premium rate (i.e., "standard" coverage only is offered, not "preferred"), while a few may let you sign on at more reasonable rates if your doctor can document that your epilepsy is well-controlled, reducing your risk of accidents or status epilepticus. Certain states require that you be accepted unless valid actuarial data (health statistics), not just assumptions about your prognosis, makes you too high of a risk according to an accepted formula.

If life insurance is part of your benefit plan at work, ask your benefits manager to work with the insurer if you are rejected. Group plans are set up to compensate for each insured person's risk factors, and your epilepsy should not count more than a coworker's pregnancy or heart murmur.

Auto insurance is also a concern for those people with seizures who drive. On auto insurance applications, you will encounter questions like, "Have you ever been treated for epilepsy?" and "Do you have a history of fainting, loss of consciousness, blackouts, seizures, or convulsions?" Insurance companies do have access to your medical records, so be sure to answer truthfully.

Auto insurance availability is also based on actuarial data: past records that show whether or not a health condition may increase a person's risk of having an auto accident. Each insurance company has its own underwriting standards, which must be based on actuarial data. Most companies offer only "standard" (higher-priced) auto insurance to persons who have had a seizure within the past five years. If you have been seizure-free for longer, you should be able to qualify for better rates, as long as you meet all other requirements for premium coverage. A few companies insure only "preferred" clients and may deny you coverage.

If you already have auto insurance and then develop epilepsy, your coverage can be revoked. You can prevent this from happening if your doctor will sign a medical waiver stating that your seizures are completely controlled on medication.

The Epilepsy Foundation suggests working with an independent insurance broker if you are buying health, life, or auto insurance on the open market. Your broker can examine plans from several different companies until one is found that meets your needs. If you are not satisfied with what you find, or if you feel you have been denied insurance unfairly, contact your state insurance commissioner for help.

Advocating for changes in the insurance and healthcare systems is a big job. Unless you want to make it your life mission, it's probably too big for any one person. But by working together, individuals can accomplish a lot.

Advocacy organizations can be the point of contact between healthcare consumers, insurers, HMOs, and public health. In the US, most insurance regulation takes place at the state level, so that's probably where the most effective efforts change will be made. There's a need for education, public advocacy, legislative action, and in some cases legal action. Patients can and should be involved in these efforts. By working closely with practitioners and with allies in the public, private, and volunteer sectors, it can happen. Even insurance companies and managed-care entities can be brought on board if they're shown the positive benefit of better-functioning people, who require much less emergency care, fewer hospitalizations, and less expensive medications. Alternative models for delivery of care are evolving, and with hard work these new systems can be both more humane and more cost-efficient.

Resources

The following list of organizations, written materials, web sites, and other resources is provided to help you do further research on partial seizure disorders, find support, and access services.

Epilepsy support and advocacy groups

Almost every country in the world has an organization devoted to advocating for and promoting the well-being of people with epilepsy. Here are the best-known national groups in the English-speaking world, each of which sponsors regional and/or local chapters.

For information about groups located elsewhere, visit the World Health Organization and the International League Against Epilepsy at *http://www.who.int/ina-ngo/ngo/ngo088.htm*.

Brainwave: The Irish Epilepsy Association
249 Crumlin Road
Dublin, Ireland
(00 353 1) 4557500

British Epilepsy Association
New Anstey House
Gate Way Dr.
Yeadon, Leeds LS19 7XY UK
Helpline (0808) 800-5050
Free fax (0808) 800-5555
epilepsy@bea.org.uk
http://www.epilepsy.org.uk

Epilepsy Association of Scotland
48 Govan Road
Glasgow, Scotland G51 1JR
(0141) 427 5225
http://www.epilepsyscotland.org.uk

Epilepsy Foundation of America (EFA)
4351 Garden City Dr.
Landover, MD 20785
(301) 459-3700 or (800) EFA-1000
Fax (301) 577-4941
webmaster@efa.org
http://www.efa.org

Epilepsy Canada/Epilepsie Canada
1470 Peel St., Suite 745
Montreal, Quebec H3A 1T1 Canada
(514) 845-7855 or (800) 860-5499
Fax (514) 845-7866
epilepsy@epilepsy.ca
http://www.epilepsy.ca

Epilepsy Concern
1282 Wynnewood Dr.
West Palm Beach, FL 33417
(407) 683-0044

Epilepsy Concern is a network of local self-help and support groups for people with epilepsy.

Epilepsy Foundation of Victoria
818-826 Burke Rd.
Camberwell, Victoria 3124 Australia
(03) 9805-9111 or (1800) 134-087
Fax (03) 9882-7159
epinet@epinet.org.au
http://www.epinet.org.au

The Epilepsy Foundation of Victoria's comprehensive web site, EpiNet, also includes links to epilepsy advocacy and support groups in other areas of Australia.

The National Society for Epilepsy
Chesham Lane
Chalfont, St. Peters
Buckinghamshire SL9 0RJ UK
Helpline 01494 601400
(01) 494 601 300
Fax: 01494 871 927
http://www.epilepsynse.org.uk

The NSE provides information about epilepsy and treatment, as well as direct services such as medical care, rehabilitation programs, residential care, and respite for caretakers.

General disability support and advocacy

The resources listed in this section provide legal information and, in some cases, practical help and advice on matters connected with disability.

Disability Rights and Education Fund
2212 6th St.
Berkeley, CA 94710
Phone/TTY: (510) 644-2555
Fax: (510) 841-8645
dredf@dredf.org
http://www.dredf.org

FindLaw
http://www.findlaw.com/01topics/36civil/disabilities.html

FindLaw has a legal research search engine, as well as a wealth of specific information about disability law.

The National Welfare Monitoring and Advocacy Partnership (NWMAP)
(202) 662-3556
info@nwmap.org
http://www.nwmap.org/index.htm

The NWMAP is a project of the Children's Defense Fund.

National Association of Protection and Advocacy Systems
900 2nd St. NE, Suite 211
Washington, DC 20002
(202) 408-9514
http://www.protectionandadvocacy.com

Every US state has a federally funded protection and advocacy system. Call this group or check its web site to find a referral to your state's P&A organization. These organizations provide legal advice, and in some cases legal representation, to people with disabilities and their family members who have disability-related needs. This may include assistance with securing federal or state benefits, advocacy in the special education system, and helping with Americans with Disabilities Act compliance issues, among other areas.

National Information Center for Children and Youth with Disabilities (NICHY)
P.O.Box 1492
Washington, DC 20013
(800) 695-0285
http://www.nichcy.org

NICHY provides free information on disabilities. Spanish-language resources are available.

National Organization of Social Security Claimants
6 Prospect St.
Midland Park, NJ 07432
(800) 432-2804
http://www.nosscr.org

National Disability Council
Caxton House, Level 4
Tothill St.
London SW1H 9NA UK
(0171) 273 5636
Fax (0171) 273 5929
Minicom (0171) 273 5579
http://www.open.gov.uk/ndc/ndchome.htm

UK Advocacy Network
Volserve House
14-18 West Bar Green
Sheffield SI 2DA UK
(0114) 272 8171

Disability Action Inc.
62 Henley Beach Road
Mile End, SA 5031 Australia
(08) 8352 8599, (800) 805 495
Fax (08) 8354 0049
TTY (08) 8352 8022
brad@disabilityaction.in-sa.com.au

Housing help for people with disabilities

Finding housing that is low-cost and constructed to accommodate disabilities can be difficult. These resources can help:

Canadian Housing Information Centre
Canada Mortgage and Housing Corporation
700 Montreal Rd.
Ottawa, Ontario K1A 0P7
(613) 748-2000
TTY (613) 748-2447
Fax (613) 748-2098
http://www.cmhc.ca

Habitat for Humanity International
Partner Service Center
121 Habitat St.
Americus, GA 31709
(912) 924-6935
publicinfo@hfhi.org
http://www.habitat.org

Habitat for Humanity is active in many areas of the world, building low-cost housing with volunteer labor and help from those who will live in the housing.

The National Disabled Persons Housing Service (HoDis)
7 Priory St.
York, YO1 6ET UK
01904 653888
Fax 01904 653999
info@hodis.org.uk
http://www.hodis.org.uk

National Home of Your Own Alliance
Institute on Disability/UAP
University of New Hampshire
7 Leavitt Lane, Suite 101
Durham, NH 03824-3522
(800) 220-8770
TDD (603) 862-4320
Fax (603) 862-0555
http://alliance.unh.edu

Opening Doors
http://www.c-c-d.org/intro_page.htm

Opening Doors is a quarterly web-based newsletter about US housing programs that benefit people with disabilities. Its site includes links to the two groups that publish it, the Technical Assistance Collaborative, Inc., and the Consortium for Citizens with Disabilities Housing Task Force.

US Department of Housing and Urban Development (HUD)
451 Seventh St. SW
Washington, DC 20414
(202) 708-4200
http://www.hud.gov

HUD finances housing for low-income and working families and administers a wide variety of housing subsidy, improvement, and construction programs.

Books and pamphlets on epilepsy

Most books about epilepsy concentrate on tonic-clonic seizures, with only a little information about partial seizures. However, even the most general of the books listed here offer excellent medical information and/or lifestyle advice, and thus should be useful to people with any type of seizure disorder:

American College of Obstetricians and Gynecologists. ACOG Educational Bulletin 231: "Seizure disorders in pregnancy." Dec. 1996. Also published in *The International Journal of Gynecology and Obstetrics*, March 1997. 56(3): 279–86.

Bennett, Thomas L. (editor). *The Neuropsychology of Epilepsy.* London: Klewer Academic Publishers/Plenum Publishing Corp., 1992.

Berent, Stanley and J. Chris Sackallares. *Psychological Disturbances in Epilepsy.* Woburn, MA: Butterworth-Heinemann Medical, 1997.

Devinsky, Orin. *A Guide to Understanding and Living with Epilepsy.* Philadelphia, PA: F. A. Davis, 1994.

Epilepsy Foundation of America. *The Legal Rights of Persons with Epilepsy.* Landover, MD: EFA, 1992.

Freeman, John M., MD. *Seizures and Epilepsy in Childhood: A Guide for Parents*, Second Edition. Baltimore, MD: Johns Hopkins University Press, 1997.

Gosselin, Kim. *Taking Seizure Disorders to School: A Story About Epilepsy.* Valley Park, MO: JayJo Books, 1998. This is an excellent book for explaining seizures to children, and it includes a section for teachers as well.

Gumnit, Robert J. *Living Well with Epilepsy, Second Edition.* New York: Demos Publications, 1997.

Hanscomb, Alice and Liz Hughes, in association with the National Center for Epilepsy. *Family Health Guide: Epilepsy.* London: Ward Lock, 1995. This is an excellent basic guide, especially for patients in the UK.

Hopkins, Anthony and Richard Appleton. *Epilepsy: The Facts*, Second Edition. Oxford: Oxford University Press, 1996.

LaPlante, Eve. *Seized: Temporal Lobe Epilepsy as a Medical, Historical, and Artistic Phenomenon.* New York: HarperCollins, 1993. This is an interesting book about temporal lobe epilepsy and its impact on the life and work of people who have it, including artists, mystics, and historical figures.

Leppik, Dr. Ilo E. *Contemporary Diagnosis and Management of the Patient with Epilepsy, Second Edition.* Newtown, PA: Handbooks in Health Care, 1996. Written for doctors but reasonably accessible for patients who want serious medical data.

Lewis, Lisa. *Special Diets for Special Kids: Implementing a Diet to Improve the Lives of Children with Autism and Related Disorders.* Arlington, Texas: Future Horizons, 1998. Includes a section on the influence of allergy, food sensitivity, and dietary changes on seizure control.

Marshall, Fiona. *Your Child and Epilepsy: Practical and Easy-to-Follow Advice.* Shaftsbury, Dorset: Element Books Ltd., 1998.

Reisner, Helen (editor). *Children with Epilepsy: A Parents Guide.* Bethesda, MD: Woodbine House, 1988.

Richard, Adrienne and Joel Reiter, MD. *Epilepsy: A New Approach*, Updated Edition. New York: Walker and Co., 1995.

Schachter, Dr. Steven C. and Donald L. Schomer, MD (editors). *The Comprehensive Evaluation and Treatment of Epilepsy: A Practical Guide.* San Diego, CA: Academic Press, 1997. Written for doctors but reasonably accessible for patients who want serious medical data.

Trimble, Michael R. (editor). *The Psychoses of Epilepsy.* New York: Raven Press, 1991.

Trimble, Michael R. and Bettina Schmidtz (editors). *Forced Normalization and Alternative Psychoses of Epilepsy.* Petersfield, UK: Wrightson Biomedical Publishing Ltd., 1998.

General medical and neurology references

These books and web sites can help you gain a better understanding of brain anatomy and brain chemistry, medical terminology, and the healthcare system. You can also use Medscape and PubMed to look up the latest clinical studies on diagnosis and treatment options.

Books

Anderson, Kenneth N., et al. (editors). *The Signet Mosby Medical Encyclopedia*, Revised Edition. New York: Signet, 1996. This book is a condensed, paperback version of *Mosby's Medical, Nursing, and Allied Health Dictionary* for health consumers.

Andreasen, Dr. Nancy C. *The Broken Brain: The Biological Revolution in Psychiatry.* New York: Harper & Row, 1984. Although it concentrates on the biology of psychiatric illness, *The Broken Brain* also does an excellent job of explaining neurochemistry concepts in accessible language.

Beers, Mark H., MD, and Robert Berkow, MD (editors). *The Merck Manual*, Seventeenth Edition. Whitehouse Station, NJ: Merck Research Laboratories, 1999. This is the standard medical reference book.

Diamond, M.C., A.B. Scheibel, and L.M. Elson. *The Human Brain Coloring Book.* New York: HarperPerennial, 1985. Believe it or not, many medical students use this book. It makes brain anatomy visual from the cellular level on up.

Keene, Nancy. *Working with Your Doctor: Getting the Healthcare You Deserve.* Sebastopol, CA: O'Reilly & Associates, 1998. This book walks you through the process of creating a partnership with your healthcare providers, in meticulous detail.

Online resources

Medscape
http://www.medscape.com

This searchable online index contains abstracts and articles from hundreds of medical journals, as well as original literature reviews and other resources.

PubMed
http://www.ncbi.nlm.nih.gov/PubMed

PubMed is a free interface for searching the MEDLINE medical database, which can help you find out about studies, medications, and more.

Genetic counseling resources

Genetic counselors have special training in helping families understand the implications of having a member diagnosed with a genetic disorder. They can explain whether these disorders will be passed on to a diagnosed person's children, and they can help you assess associated risks. They can also provide information about genetic testing for other family members.

American Board of Genetic Counseling, Inc.
9650 Rockville Pike
Bethesda, MD 20814-3998
(301) 571-1825
Fax (301) 571-1895
http://www.faseb.org/genetics/abgc/abgcmenu.htm

The ABGC credentials professionals in the field of genetic counseling and can help you find a reputable member via phone, mail, or its web site.

GeneTests
Children's Hospital and Regional Medical Center
P.O. Box 5371
Seattle, WA 98105-0371
(206) 527-5742
fax: (206) 527-5743
genetests@genetests.org
http://www.genetests.org

GeneTests is a genetic testing resource funded by the National Library of Medicine of the NIH and Maternal & Child Health Bureau of the HRSA. It provides a list of genetic research and clinical laboratories, description of genetic testing and counseling, and information for genetic professionals.

European Society of Human Genetics
Clinical Genetics Unit
Birmingham Women's Hospital
Birmingham B15 2TG UK
(44) 0-121-623-6820
esgh@esgh.org
http://www.eshg.org

Human Genetics Society of Australasia
Royal Australian College of Physicians
145 Macquarie St.
Sydney, NSW 2000 Australia
(02) 9256-5471
Fax (02) 9251-8174
hgsa@racp.edu.au
http://www.hgsa.com.au/

Medication and supplement references

There are a number of books available that list side effects, cautions, and more regarding medications. The biggest and best is the *Physicians Desk Reference* (PDR), but its price is well out of the average person's league. You may be able to find a used but recent copy at a good price, and it is available in most public libraries. The web sites listed below offer much of the same information, including effects, side effects, and risks. Some also provide manufacturing information and links to pharmaceutical companies that make specific drugs.

If your child is allergic to food dyes or to corn, wheat, and other materials used as fillers in pills, you should consult directly with the manufacturer of any medications he takes.

Books

The British National Formulary (BNF). British Medical Association and the Royal Pharmaceutical Society of Great Britain, 1999. This is the standard reference for prescribing and dispensing drugs in the UK, updated twice yearly.

Eades, Mary Dan, MD. *The Doctor's Complete Guide to Vitamins and Minerals.* New York: Dell, 1994.

Levy, Rene H., Richard Mattson, and Brian Heldrum (editors). *Antiepileptic Drugs.* New York: Raven Press, 1995. New, this book costs almost $200, but it is the most comprehensive book available on AEDs and how they work. It may be available through a local medical library.

Medical Economics Co., *Physicians Desk Reference for Herbal Medicines*, Second Edition. Montvale, NJ: Medical Economics Co., 2000.

Preston, John D., John H. O'Neal, and Mary C. Talaga. *Consumer's Guide to Psychiatric Drugs.* Oakland, CA: New Harbinger Publications, 1998.

Silverman, Harold M. (editor). *The Pill Book*, Eighth Edition. New York: Bantam Books, 1998. This is a basic paperback guide to the most commonly used medications in the US.

Sullivan, Donald. *The American Pharmaceutical Association's Guide to Prescription Drugs.* New York: Signet, 1998.

Tyler, Varro E. and Stephen Foster. *Tyler's Honest Herbal: A Sensible Guide to the Use of Herbs and Related Remedies*, Fourth Edition. Binghamton, NY: The Haworth Press, 1999.

Wilens, Timothy E., MD. *Straight Talk About Psychiatric Medications for Kids.* New York: Guilford Press, 1998.

Online resources

Canadian Drug Product Database
http://www.hc-sc.gc.ca/hpb-dgps/therapeut/htmleng/dpd.html

Dr. Bob's Psychopharmacology Tips
http://uhs.bsd.uchicago.edu/dr-bob/tips/

Federal Drug Administration (FDA)
http://www.fda.gov/cder/drug/default.htm

Official US information on new drugs and generic versions of old drugs, FDA warnings and recalls, etc., can be accessed at this web site.

The Internet Drug List
http://www.rxlist.com

MedEc Interactive/PDR.net
http://www.pdr.net
This medical info site includes a link to a Web-accessible version of the PDR.

Pharmaceutical Information Network
http://www.pharminfo.com

PharmWeb
http://www.pharmweb.net

RXmed
http://www.rxmed.com

Drug company patient assistance programs

If you do not have health insurance, or if your health insurance does not cover prescriptions, you may be eligible to receive some or all of your epilepsy medications at no charge. Most major pharmaceutical companies will accommodate requests for free or reduced price drugs; others may have reimbursement programs.

Check the package inserts for your medications to find out who makes them, and then call the patient assistance program directly. If the manufacturer's name is not listed in the following table, or if you live outside the US, talk to your pharmacist or check one of the pharmaceutical information web sites listed earlier in this appendix for more information:

Pharmaceutical Company	Phone Number
3M Pharmaceuticals	(800) 328-0255
Abbott Labs Patient Assistance Program (includes Survanta)	(800) 922-3255
American Home Products (includes Lederle)	(800) 395-9938
Amgen	(800) 272-9376
AstraZeneca (includes Ici-Stuart)	(800) 488-3247
Aventis Pharmaceuticals (includes Rhone-Poulenc Rorer, Hoecht Roussel)	(800) 207-8049
Bayer Indigent Patient Program	(800) 998-9180
Berlex	(800) 423-7539
Boehringer Ingleheim	(203) 798-4131
Bristol Myers Squibb	(800) 736-0003
Burroughs-Wellcome	(800) 722-9294
Genetech	(800) 879-4747
Glaxo, Wellcome Inc.	(800) 722-9294

Pharmaceutical Company	Phone Number
Hoffman-Larouche	(800) 526-6367
Immunex Corp.	(800) 321-4669
Janssen Pharmaceutica (includes Johnson & Johnson)	(800) 526-7736
Knoll	(800) 526-0710
Lilly Cares Program (Eli Lilly)	(800) -545-6962
Merck Human Health	(800) 672-6372
Novartis Patient Support Program (includes Sandoz, Ciba-Geigy)	(800) 257-2173
Ortho-McNeil Pharmaceuticals	(800) 682-6532
Pfizer Prescription Assistance Program (includes Parke-Davis, Warner-Lambert)	(800) 646-4455
Pharmacia Inc. (includes Upjohn)	(800) 242-7014
Procter & Gamble	(800) 448-4878
Roche Labs (includes Syntex)	(800) 285-4484
Roxane Labs	(800) 274-8651
Sanofi Winthrop	(800) 446-6267
Schering Labs	(800) 521-7157
Searle	(800) 542-2526
SmithKline Access To Care Program	(800) 546-0420 (patient requests) (215) 751-5722 (physician requests)
Solvay Patient Assistance Program	(800) 788-9277

Mail-order pharmacies

These pharmacies require a valid prescription, and some have other restrictions. When using a mail-order pharmacy outside your country, be sure to check with Customs about paperwork and permissions that may be required to import medication.

CanadaRx

http://www.canadarx.net

This is a consortium of Canadian pharmacies set up specifically to provide discounted prescriptions to US customers, although Canadians and others can use the service as well. Mail-order arrangements must be made over the Net or directly through one of the consortium members (their addresses are available on the web site).

Continental Pharmacy

PO Box 1778
Columbus, OH 43216
Phone (800) 677-4323
Fax (216) 459-0932
http://www.mimrx.com

DrugPlace.com (formerly Preferred Prescription Plan)
2201 W. Sample Road, Bldg. 9, Suite 1-A
Pompano Beach, FL 33073
Phone (954) 969-1230 or (800) 881-6325
Fax (800) 881-6990
pharmacy@drugplace.com
http://www.drugplace.com

Farmacia Rex S.R.L.
Cordoba 2401
Esq. Azcuénaga 1120
Buenos Aires, Argentina
Phone (54-1) 961-0338
Fax (54-1) 962-0153
http://www.todoservicio.com.ar/farmacia.rex/rexmenu.htm
Deeply discounted prices, and they mail anywhere.

GlobalRx
4024 Carrington Lane
Efland, NC 27243
Phone (919) 304-4278 or (800) 526-6447
Fax (919) 304-4405
info@aidsdrugs.com
http://globalrx.com
Some drugs carried by GlobalRx may not be sent to US customers.

Masters Marketing Company, Ltd.
Masters House
5 Sandridge Close
Harrow, Middlesex HA1 1TW UK
Phone (011) 44-181-424-9400
Fax (011) 44-181-427-1994
mmc@mastersint.com
http://business.fortunecity.com/ingram/858/index.HTM
Carries a limited selection of European and American pharmaceuticals.

No Frills Pharmacy
1510 Harlan Dr.
Bellevue, NE 68005
Phone (800) 485-7423
Fax (402) 682-9899
refill@nofrillspharmacy.com
http://www.nofrillspharmacy.com

Peoples Pharmacy
http://www.peoplesrx.com
This Austin, Texas-based chain provides Net-only mail-order service and can compound medications as well.

Pharmacy Direct
3 Coal St.
Silverwater, NSW 2128 Australia
Phone (02) 9648-8888 or (1300) 656-245
Fax (02) 9648 8999 or (1300) 656 329
pharmacy@pharmacydirect.com.au
http://www.pharmacydirect.com.au

You must have a prescription from an Australian doctor to use this mail-order service.

The Pharmacy Shop (also known as Drugs By Mail)
5007 N. Central
Phoenix, AZ 85012
Phone (602) 274-9956 or (800) 775-6888
Fax (602) 241-0104
sales@drugsbymail.com
http://www.pharmacyshop.com or *http://www.drugsbymail.com*

The Pharmacy Shop is one of the mail-order vendors that will waive your medication co-pay, if you have the right insurance plan.

Stadtlanders Pharmacy
600 Penn Center Blvd.
Pittsburgh, PA 15235-5810
(800) 238-7828
enroll@stadtlander.com
http://stadtlander.com

Stadtlanders Pharmacy has a stellar reputation in the disability community.

Victoria Apotheke (Victoria Pharmacy)
c/o Dr. C. Egloff, PhD
PO Box CH-8021
Zurich, Switzerland
Fax (01) 221-23-22 (Europe) or (011) 411-221-23-22 (US)
Phone (01) 211-24-32 (Europe) or (011) 411-211-24-32 (US)
victoriaapotheke@access.ch
http://www.access.ch/victoria_pharmacy

Patient travel assistance programs

Most airlines accept donations of unused frequent flyer miles and use these gifts to subsidize air travel for patients in need of treatment or other charitable purposes. You can contact airlines directly or try one of the programs listed below. You may also want to check with charitable organizations such as the United Way or Salvation Army, many of which are recipients of the airlines' mileage and gift certificate donations.

AirLifeLine
(800) 446-1231
http://www.airlifeline.org

This group of volunteer pilots provides transportation aboard private planes to patients traveling for diagnostic or treatment services.

Delta SkyWish Program
(800) 892-2757, x285
http://electronicvalley.org/vuw/skywish.html

This program, which is administered through the United Way of America, provides medical travel assistance to people with life-threatening illnesses.

Continental Care Force
(281) 261-6626

Miracle Flights For Kids
2756 N. Green Valley Parkway, Suite 115
Green Valley, NV 89014-0497
(702) 261-0494
Fax (702) 261-0497
http://www.miracleflights.com

This group provides flights for children and families traveling for medical help. Private and corporate jets flown by volunteer pilots are used, although patients are occasionally placed on commercial flights.

National Patient Air Transport Hotline
Mercy Medical Airlift
4620 Haygood Rd., Suite 8
Virginia Beach, VA 93455
Fax (757) 318-9107
(800) 296-1217

The National Patient Air Transport Hotline makes referrals to TWA Operation Liftoff, AirLifeLine, and other programs.

Wings of Freedom
(407) 363-1991

This service negotiates with commercial airlines for low-cost tickets.

Patient lodging assistance programs

If you or your child will be traveling to a major medical center for treatment or surgery, call the hospital or clinic's social worker in advance for information about free or low-cost local housing options. They can put you in touch with the nearest Ronald McDonald House or similar programs and advise you on hotels that offer reduced rates to visiting patients and their families. Hostels are another option for low-cost housing; see *http://www.hostels.com* or more information. In some facilities, parents are able to spend the night in their child's room at no extra charge. You can also call:

National Association of Hospitality Houses
(800) 542-9730

The ketogenic diet

The ketogenic diet should only be undertaken as part of a carefully supervised medical treatment program. These resources can help you with information, recipes, and support to make the experience easier.

Books

Brake, Dennis, and Cynthia Brake. *The Ketogenic Cookbook*. Gilman, CT: Pennycorner Press, 1997.

Freeman, John M., MD. *The Epilepsy Diet Treatment: An Introduction to the Ketogenic Diet*, Second Edition. New York: Demos Vermande, 1996.

Online resources

Ketogenic Diet site
Packard Children's Hospital
Stanford University Medical Center
http://www.stanford.edu/group/ketodiet

Family Village Ketogenic diet site
http://www.familyvillage.wisc.edu/general/ketogeni.htm

This web site includes links to online discussion groups, a printed newsletter, basic ketogenic diet information, and more.

Newsletters for people with seizure disorders

Most national and regional epilepsy organizations also publish newsletters that are sent to all members. Many epilepsy treatment centers also have informative newsletters for patients and other interested persons.

Epilepsy Quarterly
http://www.epifellows.com/EQRT/EQTOC.html

This online newsletter, in Adobe Acrobat format, provides the latest information from epilepsy research.

Epilepsy Wellness Newsletter
1462 W. 5th Ave.
Eugene, OR 97402

This newsletter accents alternative approaches to epilepsy treatment.

Online resources for people with seizure disorders

See also the web sites for the epilepsy support and advocacy groups listed earlier in this appendix.

The Epilepsy Connection
http://www.epilepsy-connect.org/index.shtml

Epilepsy International
http://www.epiworld.com/

Information about epilepsy, available in English and Spanish.

EPILEPSY-L
http://home.ease.lsoft.com/Archives/Epilepsy-L.html

EPILEPSY-L is an email discussion group for people with seizure disorders and their family members. You can subscribe or read the archives at the web site above. If you don't have web access, email your request to subscribe to this address: *epilepsy-l-request@home.ease.lsoft.com*.

Neurology Webforums at Massachusetts General Hospital
http://neuro-mancer.mgh.harvard.edu/cgi-bin/Ultimate.cgi

These bulletin board–style forums allow you to post or answer questions and to read what others have written. Several epilepsy variants and related topics have a discussion group here, and there are live discussions at a related site as well.

Diagnostic centers

This section lists several of the best-known university-affiliated and private programs in the US with special expertise in seizure disorders. This is by no means a comprehensive list. Persons outside the US should contact their national epilepsy association for information about the best resources in their area.

Adult Epilepsy Center/Child Epilepsy Center
Washington University School of Medicine
Department of Neurology
Washington University Medical Center
St. Louis, MO 63110
(314) 454-2692 or (314) 362-4838
http://www.neuro.wustl.edu/epilepsy/index.html

Blue Bird Circle Clinic for Pediatric Neurology
Baylor College of Medicine
Dept. of Neurology
6501 Fannin St.
Houston, TX 77030
(713) 790-5046
Fax (713) 793-1313
http://www.bcm.tmc.edu/neurol/struct/blueb/blueb1.html

The Blue Bird Clinic specializes in treating children and maintains a special clinic for children with Rett syndrome.

Epilepsy Center
5405 Southwyck Blvd.
Toledo, OH 43614
(419) 867-5950 or (800) 589-5958
epilepsycenter@solarstop.net
http://www.epilepsycenter.com

Johns Hopkins Epilepsy Center
Johns Hopkins University
School of Medicine
720 Rutland Ave.
Baltimore, MD 21205
(410) 955-3184
http://www.neuro.jhmi.edu/epilepsy/Epilepsy.html

MGH Epilepsy Service
Massachusetts General Hospital
15 Parkman St., Suite 835
Boston, MA 02114
(617) 726-2000
http://neuro-oas.mgh.harvard.edu/epilepsy/

Mid-Atlantic Regional Epilepsy Center
Medical College of Pennsylvania Hospital
300 Henry Ave.
Philadelphia, PA 19129
(215) 842-6000
http://www.auhs.edu/medschool/depts/neurology/epilepsy.htm

Minnesota Comprehensive Epilepsy Care Program (MINCEP)
775 Wayzata Blvd., #255
Minneapolis, MN 55416
(612) 525-2400
Fax (612) 525-1560

National Association of Epilepsy Centers
5775 Wayzata Boulevard
Suite 200
Minneapolis, Minnesota 55416
(612) 525-4511

Rush Epilepsy Center
Rush-Presbyterian-St. Luke's Medical Center
1653 W. Congress Parkway
Chicago, IL 60612
(312) 942-5939
http://www.campus.rpslmc.edu/patients/children/services/specialties/neurological/epilepsy. html

Stanford Comprehensive Epilepsy Center (for adults)
Stanford University Medical Center
300 Pasteur Dr., A343
Stanford, CA 94305-5235
(650) 725-6648 or (650) 723-6469 for appointments
Fax (650) 725-7459
http://www.stanford.edu/group/neurology

University of Washington Regional Epilepsy Center
325 9th Ave., Box 359745
Seattle, WA 98104-2499
(800) 374-3627
Fax (206) 731-4409
http://elliott.hmc.washington.edu/index.html

Special education

These books and web sites will help you gain an enhanced understanding of special education law so that you can advocate for your child during the IFSP and IEP process.

Books

Anderson, Winifred, Stephen Chitwood, and Dierdre Hayden. *Negotiating the Special Education Maze: A Guide for Parents and Teachers*, Third Edition. Rockville, MD: Woodbine House, 1997. Well-written and very complete, this new edition includes information on the changes wrought by IDEA '97.

Cutler, Barbara Coyne. *You, Your Child, and "Special" Education: A Guide to Making the System Work.* Baltimore, MD: Paul H. Brookes Publishing Co., 1993. An uppity guide to fighting the system on your child's behalf.

Online resources

Advocating for the Child
http://www.crosswinds.net/washington-dc/~advocate/index.html

Maintained by the mother of neurologically challenged children, this site is an all-purpose guide to advocating for your child's educational rights in the US. It's information-rich, with great links and lots of inspiration.

The Special Ed Advocate/Wrightslaw
http://www.wrightslaw.com

This site contains the actual text of special education laws, information on the latest court battles, and answers to your special education questions.

Special Education and Disabilities Resources
http://www.educ.drake.edu/rc/sp_ed_top.html

US information and links on special education law, assistive technology, and related topics.

Learning Disabilities Online
http://www.ldonline.org

Covers all aspects of special education and learning difficulties.

Sibling issues

In families coping with childhood disability or illness, the non-affected siblings also experience stresses and may require special help. These books and web sites attempt to address sibling issues.

Meyer, Donald, and Patricia Vadasy, *Living with a Brother or Sister with Special Needs*. Seattle, WA: University of Washington Press, 1996.

Meyer, Donald, editor. *Views from Our Shoes: Growing up with a Brother or Sister with Special Needs*. Rockville, MD: Woodbine House, 1997.

SibShops/Sibling Support Project
Children's Hospital and Medical Center
PO Box 5371, CL-09
Seattle, WA 98105
(206) 368-4911
Fax (206) 368-4816
http://www.chmc.org/departmt/sibsupp/sibshoppage.htm

SibShops are special support groups for children dealing with a sibling's disability. This site provides information on SibShops and related topics, and it can help you find a SibShop program in your area.

Healthcare and insurance

Healthcare and insurance can be difficult issues for people with disabilities. The following resources include information about navigating bureaucracies for better care, and obtaining needed services and coverage.

Beckett, Julie. *Health Care Financing: A Guide for Families*, National Maternal and Child Health Resource Center. (Order from: NMCHRC, Law Building, University of Iowa, Iowa City, IA 52242; (319) 335-9073.) This overview of the healthcare financing system includes advocacy strategies for families and information about public health insurance in the US.

Larson, Georgianna, and Judith Kahn. *Special Needs/Special Solutions: How to Get Quality Care for a Child with Special Health Needs*. St. Paul, MN: Life Line Press, 1991.

Neville, Kathy. "Strategic Insurance Negotiation: An Introduction to Basic Skills for Families and Community Mental Health Workers" (Order from: CAPP/NPRC Project, Federation for Children with Special Needs, 95 Berkeley St., Suite 104, Boston, MA 02116.) Single copies of this pamphlet are available at no cost.

Insure Kids Now
Children's Heath Insurance Program (CHIPs)
(877) 543-7669
http://www.insurekidsnow.gov

CHIPs is a federal program that encourages US states to establish health insurance programs for uninsured children, based on Medicaid waivers. This site includes information about and links to state programs.

National Association of Insurance Commissioners (NAIC)
444 National Capitol St. NW, Suite 309
Washington, DC 20001
(202) 624-7790

Call NAIC to locate your state insurance commissioner, who can tell you about health insurance regulations in your state regarding seizure disorders.

Seizure Diary

You can reproduce the journal on the following page to help you keep track of lifestyle issues that may affect your seizures, or you may want to adapt it based on personal seizure triggers already identified.

The category of stressors is provided for noting anything that might cause additional physical or mental stress. Examples of typical stressors that may affect seizure type and frequency include premenstrual symptoms and menstruation, illness, job or personal emotional stress, the use of non-prescription drugs or alcohol, and any other factor that you suspect may influence your symptoms.

Time	Sleep	Medication	Foods	Stressors	Seizures and Other Symptoms
12:00 am					
1:00 am					
2:00 am					
3:00 am					
4:00 am					
5:00 am					
6:00 am					
7:00 am					
8:00 am					
9:00 am					
10:00 am					
11:00 am					
12:00 pm					
1:00 pm					
2:00 pm					
3:00 pm					
4:00 pm					
5:00 pm					
6:00 pm					
7:00 pm					
8:00 pm					
9:00 pm					
10:00 pm					
11:00 pm					

Glossary

This list of epilepsy-related terms is by no means complete, but it should help people coping with a new diagnosis or confusing paperwork. Some of these terms, like petit mal seizure, are considered outdated; others are used more often in the UK than in the US, or vice versa.

All of the specific medical disorders involving seizures defined here, such as Landau-Kleffner syndrome and Rett syndrome, are exceedingly rare. They include serious, and usually quite obvious, symptoms apart from the seizures themselves. Parents of children who have partial seizures but not the other distinctive symptoms of such disorders need not worry; we list them mainly to define terms that you may hear about in relation to seizures, especially seizures in childhood.

Abdominal seizure
> A seizure that includes stomach pain or other symptoms related to the digestive system, such as nausea, vomiting, or flatulence. See also autonomic phenomena.

Abreactive seizure
> A seizure that occurs in response to emotional stress.

Absence seizure
> A seizure characterized by temporary loss of connection with events in the outside world: "The lights are on, but there's nobody home." Absence seizures almost always start in childhood and often disappear in early adulthood. See also absence seizure, typical; absence seizure, atypical; generalized seizure.

Absence seizure, atypical
> A seizure featuring sudden impairment of consciousness, possibly accompanied by a blank facial expression, and with associated movements or behaviors. The most common of these are simple automatisms, such as lip-smacking, eye-batting, or a jerking arm.

Absence seizure, typical
> A seizure featuring sudden impairment of consciousness, possibly accompanied by a blank facial expression but without any associated movements. Despite the name, typical absence seizures are actually less common than atypical ones.

Absence status
> The condition of having a near-continuous series of absence seizures. See also status epilepticus.

Acquired epileptic aphasia
> See Landau-Kleffner syndrome.

Aicardi syndrome
  A rare, severe, genetic seizure disorder that begins with infantile spasms, and affects only girls. A part of the brain called the corpus callosum is missing, and there are abnormalities in the retina of the eye.

Akinetic fall
  A sudden loss of muscle control.

Angelman's syndrome
  A rare genetic disorder characterized by seizures, including gelastic seizures, developmental delay, and a unique facial appearance.

Astatic seizure
  See atonic seizure.

Atonic seizure
  A seizure in which the body loses muscle tone, becoming floppy and uncontrollable. A standing person may fall down; a sitting person may slump over.

Aura
  A simple partial seizure. This term is usually used to indicate a simple partial seizure that occurs before a complex partial or tonic-clonic seizure.

Automatism
  An automatic movement occurring during a seizure, without the patient's awareness. Usually the patient cannot remember these movements later. Automatisms are normally simple movements, like pulling at your shirt, but can include complex behaviors that look voluntary, such as bouncing a ball.

Autonomic phenomena
  Symptoms occurring during a seizure due to aberrant activity of the autonomic nervous system. Autonomic phenomena can include sudden pupil dilation, facial paleness or flushing, drooling, stomach pain, and loss of urinary control.

Benign occipital epilepsy
  See childhood epilepsy with occipital paroxysms.

Benign familial neonatal seizures
  Seizures occurring in an otherwise normal newborn baby for no apparent reason, but with a family history of such seizures. The seizures end after the newborn period without harmful consequences.

Benign neonatal convulsions
  See benign neonatal idiopathic seizures.

Benign neonatal idiopathic seizures
  Seizures occurring in an otherwise normal newborn baby for no known reason and ending after the newborn period without harmful consequences.

Benign partial seizure of childhood
  See Rolandic epilepsy.

Benign Rolandic epilepsy of childhood
  See Rolandic epilepsy.

Catamenial epilepsy
  Epilepsy in which the menstrual cycle affects the timing and severity of seizure activity.

Childhood epilepsy with occipital paroxysms

A seizure disorder characterized by partial seizures involving the occipital lobe, and therefore presenting with visual disturbances (hallucinations, seeing lights, etc.) as its main syndrome. Some patients experience migraine-like headaches and/or nausea after the seizure. Also known as Gastaut syndrome—not to be confused with Lennox-Gastaut syndrome.

Complex partial seizure

A partial seizure that affects two or more areas of the brain, but not the entire brain. They almost always involve the temporal or frontal lobe.

Complex partial status epilepticus

The condition of having a series of complex partial seizures. Also called continuous partial epilepsy. See also status epilepticus.

Continuous spike-wave epilepsy

As the name indicates, a seizure disorder characterized by a specific type of spike-wave pattern on an EEG. This pattern appears when the patient is asleep, but may not be present during waking hours.

Cryptogenic epilepsy

Epilepsy for which the cause is not known but for which a diagnosable physical cause is suspected.

Drop attack

See atonic seizure.

Encephalitis

Inflammation of the brain. Encephalitis can be due to infection of the brain by microorganisms that somehow pass through the protective blood-brain barrier, such as one of the herpes viruses, or by an autoimmune reaction, as in Rasmussen's encephalitis. Encephalitis can cause brain damage that causes seizures later on, or it can cause seizures directly.

Febrile seizures

Seizures associated with a high fever. These are common in infants and rarely a cause for future concern.

Focal cortical seizure

See partial seizure.

Focal-local seizure

See partial seizure.

Frontal lobe epilepsy

A seizure disorder where the primary focus is in the frontal lobe. It resembles temporal lobe epilepsy, except that the seizures are shorter, more frequent, and often occur in clusters; any automatisms are more likely to involve the legs; there is very likely to be uninhibited and possibly aggressive or sexually inappropriate behavior during the seizure; and there is less likelihood of confusion after the seizure.

Gelastic seizure

A seizure that includes uncontrollable laughter. Gelastic seizures often happen during sleep.

Generalized seizure
> Any type of seizure that affects the entire brain, including absence, myoclonic, atonic, and tonic-clonic seizures.

Grand mal seizures
> See tonic-clonic seizure.

Hypoglycemic seizure
> A seizure whose trigger is a sudden drop in blood sugar. This type of seizure is most common in people with poorly controlled diabetes, and it can usually be controlled by lifestyle change alone.

Idiopathic epilepsy
> Epilepsy for which the cause is not known.

Idiopathic partial seizure
> See Rolandic epilepsy.

Ictal
> During a seizure.

Infantile spasms
> A severe seizure disorder affecting a child under age two and often associated with developmental delay. The seizures are tonic or myoclonic, often occur in clusters, and frequently happen just as the infant is waking up or falling asleep. A hypsarrythmic pattern is seen on an EEG. Infantile spasms are blessedly rare; they are hard to control with current medication and generally have a poor outcome. Also known as salaam seizures or West syndrome. Aicardi syndrome is a specific disorder that involves infantile spasms.

Interictal
> Between seizures.

Interictal personality syndrome
> Some older neurology books refer to certain unusual behaviors and sensations by this or similar terms. Today we know that most of these phenomena, which include hypergraphia (incessant writing), sexual disturbances, and a stronger than average interest in philosophical or religious matters, derive from disturbances in areas of the brain affected by seizures, particularly the temporal lobe.

Jacksonian seizure
> See simple partial seizure.

Janz syndrome
> See juvenile myoclonic epilepsy.

Juvenile absence epilepsy
> Repeated absence seizures that start during puberty or the teen years.

Juvenile myoclonic epilepsy
> A seizure disorder characterized by myoclonic jerks, usually of the hands, arms, or torso, that starts around puberty or in the teen years. Myoclonic seizures are especially common right after waking in the morning and may also be set off by sleep deprivation or alcohol use. Unlike many other forms of childhood-onset epilepsy, JME almost always continues into adulthood.

Landau Kleffner syndrome

A seizure disorder that results in loss of speech (aphasia) some time after eighteen months of age. It is twice as common in males and may result in autism-like symptoms.

Lennox-Gastaut syndrome

A disorder starting in childhood that may feature many different types of seizures, especially tonic seizures, usually accompanied by developmental delay. Its cause is unknown, and it is extremely difficult to treat since many patients do not respond to the usual antiseizure drugs. On an EEG, patients with Lennox-Gastaut syndrome have a characteristic slow spike-and-wave pattern.

Lesion

An area of brain damage, or scar. A lesion in the brain can be a seizure focus and can often be seen using brain-scanning technology, such as an MRI.

Myoclonic jerk

Uncontrollable jerking of a muscle group, resulting in a twitching limb or head, or even a whole-body jerk. The person will not be conscious during this movement, and if standing, she may lose her balance and fall. Myoclonic seizures are most common just after waking and are usually quite brief. Myoclonic seizures should not be confused with a myoclonic twitch—a common, harmless, contraction of a small muscle, such as one of the muscles near the eye—or with the repeated physical movements known as tics. A person with a tic disorder, such as Tourette syndrome, or a myoclonic twitch does not lose consciousness during his jerky movements.

Myoclonic seizure

See myoclonic jerk.

Musicogenic seizure

A seizure triggered by music or during which the person hears music.

Necrosis

Tissue death. Dead tissue in the brain can be a seizure focus. The brain's natural tendency is to surround any area of necrosis with scar tissue (see sclerosis).

Neonatal seizures

Seizures occurring in a newborn infant. Neonatal seizures are often a sign of serious brain injury before, during, or just after birth. They can be caused by brain infection and inflammation (see encephalitis), brain damage or malformation, oxygen deprivation (nuchal cord at birth, anoxia), or a metabolic disorder.

Nocturnal seizure

A seizure that occurs while the patient is sleeping.

Partial motor seizure

A partial seizure that results in uncontrolled physical movements. See also partial seizures.

Partial seizure

A seizure that affects only one area of the brain. See also partial motor seizures, simple partial seizures, and complex partial seizures.

Periictal

Before a seizure.

Petit mal seizure
See absence seizure.

Photosensitive epilepsy
Seizures triggered by exposure to certain types of light. Some people with photosensitive epilepsy are extraordinarily sensitive even to natural light in normal amounts. Most people with photosensitive epilepsy are sensitive only to certain types of light, such as flickering fluorescent tubes or strobe lights.

Postictal
After a seizure. Postictal confusion refers to feelings of disorientation or altered mood that may happen after a seizure.

Preictal
Before a seizure.

Prodromal
Before a seizure. The term prodrome is sometimes used to describe an aura that occurs before a tonic-clonic seizure. See also aura.

Pseudoseizure
Technically, a seizure-like episode not caused by abnormal discharge of neurons in the brain. Realistically, events labeled as pseudoseizures range from deliberate attempts to act as though one is having seizures to get attention, to the seizure-like effects of other illnesses, to seizures that simply cannot be picked up with current monitoring equipment. A common example of a pseudoseizure is convulsive syncope, fainting with convulsion-like body movements. Sometimes called psychogenic seizures, factitious (false) seizures, or non-epileptic seizures.

Psychomotor seizures
See complex partial seizures.

Pyknolepsy
A seizure disorder starting in childhood and characterized by repeated absence seizures. It usually disappears by adulthood, and these absence seizures are generally easily controlled through medication and lifestyle adjustments.

Pyknoleptic petit mal seizure
See pyknolepsy, absence seizure.

Rasmussen's encephalitis
A syndrome of brain inflammation characterized by seizures and linked to an autoimmune response to part of the glutamate neurotransmitter.

Rett syndrome
A condition cased by a genetic mutation on the X chromosome, characterized by slow growth, small head (microcephaly), mental retardation, autism-like symptoms, a characteristic hand-wringing movement, and muscle tremors. About 80 percent of people with Rett syndrome also have epilepsy. It is currently believed that male fetuses with the Rett gene cannot survive, so all currently diagnosed patients are female.

Rolandic epilepsy
A seizure disorder that starts in childhood and usually disappears in the teen years. The seizures usually occur at night and are almost always partial motor seizures. On an EEG, a spike focus is seen in the midtemporal-central area of the brain, near a brain structure called the central gyrus of Rolando. The usual

treatment for benign Rolandic epilepsy is simply observation. If the seizures seem to cause sleep disturbance or cognitive problems, medication may be tried until the child is older.

Salaam seizures
See infantile spasms.

Sclerosis
Scar tissue. In the brain, sclerosis can be a seizure focus.

Secondary epilepsy
See symptomatic epilepsy.

Simple partial seizure
A seizure that affects only one area of the brain, without loss of consciousness.

Status epilepticus
An extremely prolonged seizure, or the condition of one seizure following upon another. This is a potentially deadly event if the seizures are generalized. See also absence status, complex partial status epilepticus.

Stereotypies
Repetitive, purposeless, uncontrollable movements that occur during a partial or absence seizure. Typical stereotypies include mouth movements and minor arm or leg twitching.

Sturge-Weber syndrome
See vascular malformation.

Sylvan seizures
See Rolandic epilepsy.

Symptomatic epilepsy
Epilepsy for which the cause is known. Common and uncommon causes of symptomatic epilepsy include high fever, head injury, brain infection, brain tumor, and structural differences in the brain.

Temporal lobe epilepsy
A seizure disorder in which the primary focus is in the temporal lobe. Often abbreviated as TLE, temporal lobe epilepsy is characterized by specific types of psychic and sensory disturbances. The seizures usually last from one to three minutes and rarely occur in clusters; any automatisms usually affect the face, arms, and/or hands. After the seizure the patient may feel confused or disoriented.

Tonic seizure
A seizure in which the body becomes rigid and stiff, without convulsions as in a tonic-clonic seizure, but with loss of consciousness.

Tonic seizure, asymmetric
A tonic seizure that affects primarily muscles on one side of the body.

Tonic seizure, axial
A tonic seizure that starts in the neck muscles and progresses to stiffen the facial muscles as well. The respiratory and stomach muscles often stiffen up next.

Tonic seizure, axorhizomelic
A tonic seizure that starts like an axial tonic seizure, but then spreads to the shoulders and arms.

Tonic seizure, global

A tonic seizure in which the muscle stiffness extends to the arms and sometimes the legs. The person's arms flex and are pulled up toward the chest. If the legs are affected, the person may fall.

Tonic-clonic seizure

A seizure in which the rigid tonic state is followed by the jerking clonic state, usually repeatedly. This produces a convulsion, in which the person may be writhing on the floor and will lose consciousness. After the seizure the person may feel very tired, confused, and sore.

Tuberous sclerosis

A syndrome characterized by the growth of non-cancerous, tumor-like growths inside the brain. The presence of these tubers can cause seizures as well as mood swings and autism-like symptoms.

Tumor

An abnormal growth, usually of soft tissue but sometimes of bone or other tissue. When a tumor occurs in the brain it can cause seizures, whether it is benign (non-cancerous) or cancerous. This is a rare cause for seizures.

Vascular malformation

A malformed blood vessel or vessels. When a vascular malformation occurs in the brain, seizures may result. This is a rare cause for seizures, and when it occurs there are usually other more obvious physical signs and symptoms of a general birth defect syndrome, such as Sturge-Weber syndrome.

West syndrome

See infantile spasms.

Notes

Chapter 1, *Introduction to Partial Seizure Disorders*

1. Jacqueline A. French, MD, and Norman Elanty, MD. "Emerging Strategies for Early Seizure Control." *Neurology Treatment Updates*, Medscape Inc., 1999: *http://www.medscape.com/medscape/Neurology/TreatmentUpdate/1999/tu01/public/toc-tu01.html*.

Chapter 2, *Diagnosis*

1. Ilo Leppik, MD. *Contemporary Diagnosis and Management of the Patient with Epilepsy*, Newtown, PA: Associates in Medical Marketing Co, Inc., 1996: 47.
2. Mark Cote, DO, et al. "Tc99m-HMPAO for the Detection of a Seizure Focus: Partial Complex Seizures/Temporal Lobe Epilepsy." United States Army Medical Command, 1995: *http://www.mamc.amedd.army.mil/WILLIAMS/NucMed/CNS/Seizure%20imaging/Seizure%20imaging.html*.
3. R. A. Bronen, et al. "Refractory epilepsy: Comparison of MR imaging, CT, and Histopathologic Findings in 177 patients," *Radiology*, 1996. 201: 97–105.
4. S. S. Spencer. "The Relative Contributions of MRI, SPECT, and PET Imaging in Epilepsy," *Epilepsia*: 1994. 35: S72.
5. P. Szepetowski and A. P. Monaco. "Recent Progress in the Genetics of Human Epilepsies," *Neurogenetics,* March 1998. 1(3): 153–163.
6. Linda R. Thomsen, MSN. "Nonepileptic Seizures: Avoid Misdiagnosis and Long-term Morbidity." *Clinician Reviews*, 1998. 8(3): *http://www.medscape.com/CPG/ClinReviews/1998/v08.n03/c0803.02.thom/c0803.02.thom.html*.
7. Bizhan Aarabi, MD, et al. "Prognostic Factors in the Occurrence of Posttraumatic Epilepsy After Penetrating Head Injury Suffered During Military Service," *Neurosurgical Focus,* Jan. 2000. 8(1).
8. J. L. Cummings. *Clinical Neuropsychiatry*. Orlando, FL: Grue/Stratton, 1985.
9. "Critical Issues in the Use of Anti-Epileptic Drugs: Special Issues in Elderly Patients With Seizures." *Neurology Treatment Updates*, Medscape, 2000: *http://www.medscape.com/medscape/Neurology/TreatmentUpdate/2000/tu04/tu04-03.html*.
10. Pierre Tariot and Anton Porsteinsson. Presentation to 6th International Conference on Alzheimer's Disease and Related Disorders. 1998: Summarized at *http://www.rochester.edu/pr/releases/med/alz98.htm*.
11. Christopher S. Ogilvy, MD, and Stephen B. Tatter, MD, PhD. "Central Nervous System Vascular Malformations: A Patient's Guide." *http://brain.mgh.harvard.edu:100/vascintr.htm*.
12. Ruth Ottman and Richard Lipton. "Comorbidity of Migraine and Epilepsy," *Neurology*, 1994. 44: 2105–10.

13. M. V. Lambert and M. M. Robertson. "Depression in Epilepsy: Etiology, Phenomenology, and Treatment," *Epilepsia* 1999. 40 (Supplement 10): S21–47.

Chapter 3, *Living with Partial Seizure Disorders*

1. World Health Organization. "Epilepsy: Social Consequences and Economic Aspects," WHO Fact Sheet N166, June 1997.
2. Gus Baker, et al. "The Stigma of Epilepsy: A European Perspective," *Epilepsia*, 2000. 41: 98.
3. Jamie Dalrymple and John Appleby. "Cross Sectional Study of Reporting of Epileptic Seizures to General Practitioners," *British Medical Journal* 320, Jan. 8, 2000. 320: 94–7.
4. "With Proper Care, Successful Pregnancy Likely in Women with Epilepsy," *Drugs & Therapy Perspectives,* 2000. 15(4): 5–8: *http://www.medscape.com/adis/DTP/2000/v15.n04/dtp1504.02/dtp1504.02-01.html.*
5. E. B. Samren, et al. "Antiepileptic Drug Regimens and Major Congenital Abnormalities in the Offspring." *Annals of Neurology,* November 1999. 46(5): 739–46.
6. Ibid.
7. Ibid.

Chapter 5, *Medical Interventions*

1. Solomon Moshe, MD. "Neuroprotection and Epilepsy." *Neurology Treatment Updates*, Medscape Inc., 2000: *http://www.medscape.com/medscape/Neurology/TreatmentUpdate/2000/tu01/public/toc-tu01.html.*
2. Ibid.
3. Ibid.
4. F. Monaco and A. Cicolin. "Interactions Between Anticonvulsant and Psychoactive Drugs," *Epilepsia,* 1999. 40 S10: S71–S76.
5. Orrin Devinsky, MD. *A Guide to Understanding and Living with Epilepsy*. Philadelphia, PA: F. A. Davis Co., 1994: 124–39.

Chapter 6, *Other Interventions*

1. Tim Betts, MD. Research at the University of Birmingham epilepsy clinic, as reported by the British Epilepsy Association.
2. Adrienne Richard and Joel Reiter, MD. *Epilepsy: A New Approach*. New York: Walker and Co., 1995: 193.
3. A. O. Ogunmekan and P. A. Hwang. "A Randomized, Double-Blind, Placebo-Controlled, Clinical Trial of D-alpha-tocopheryl Acetate (Vitamin E), as Add-on Therapy, for Epilepsy in Children," *Epilepsia*, Jan.–Feb. 1989. 30(1): 84–9.
4. U. Moslet, and E. S. Hansen. "A Review of Vitamin K, Epilepsy and Pregnancy," *Acta Neurologica Scandinavica,* 1992. 85: 39–43.
5. F. B. Gibberd, A. Nicholls, and M. G. Wright. "The Influence of Folic Acid on the Frequency of Epileptic Attacks," *European Journal of Clinical Pharmacology,* 1981. 19: 57–60.
6. L. Guidolin, A. Vignoli, and R. Canger. "Worsening in Seizure Frequency and Severity in Relation to Folic Acid Administration," *European Journal of Neurology,* 1998. 5: 301–3.

7. D. M. Mock and M. E. Dyken. "Biotin Catabolism Is Accelerated in Adults Receiving Long-term Therapy with Anticonvulsants," *Neurology*, 1997. 49: 1444–7.

8. D. M. Mock, et al. "Disturbances in Biotin Metabolism in Children Undergoing Long-term Anticonvulsant Therapy," *Journal of Pediatric Gastroenterology and Nutrition*, 1998. 26: 245–50.

9. J. P. Van Wouwe. "Carnitine Deficiency During Valproic Acid Treatment," *International Journal of Vitamin and Nutrition Research*, 1995. 65: 211–4.

10. J. V. Murphy, K. M. Marquardt, and A. L. Shug. "Valproic Acid Associated with Abnormalities of Carnitine Metabolism," *Lancet*, 1985. 1: 820–1.

11. P. Monteleone, et al. "Suppression of Nocturnal Plasma Melatonin Levels by Evening Administration of Sodium Valproate in Healthy Humans," *Biological Psychiatry*, 1997. 41: 336–41.

12. J. Gleitz, et al. "Anticonvulsant Action of Kavain Estimated From Its Properties on Stimulated Synaptosomes and Na+ Channel Receptor Sites," *European Journal of Pharmacology*, 1996. 315(1): 89–97.

13. A. P. Simopoulos. "Omega-3 Fatty Acids in Health and Disease and in Growth and Development," *American Journal of Clinical Nutrition*, 1991. 54(3): 438–63.

14. Andrew L. Stoll, MD, et al. "Omega-3 Fatty Acids in Bipolar Disorder: A Preliminary Double-Blind, Placebo-Controlled Trial," *Archives of General Psychiatry*, May 1999. 56(5): 407–12.

15. Andrew L. Stoll, MD. "Omega-3 Fatty Acid User Guide." 1998. [Order from: Psychopharmacology Research Laboratory, McLean Hospital, 115 Mill St., Belmont, MA 02478].

16. P. R. Camfield, et al. "Aspartame Exacerbates EEG Spike-wave Discharge in Children with Generalized Absence Epilepsy: A Double-Blind Controlled Study," *Neurology*, May 1992. 42(5): 1000–3.

17. Carl Stafstrom and Susan Spencer. "The Ketogenic Diet: A Therapy in Search of an Explanation," *Neurology*, 2000. 54: 282–3.

18. J. P. Ferroir, et al. "Epilepsy, Cerebral Calcifications and Celiac Disease," *Revista del Neurologia*, June 1997. 153(5): 354–6.

19. L. Francetti, et al. "Oral Hygiene in Subjects Treated with Diphenylhydantoin: Effects of a Professional Program," *Prevenzione e Assistenza Dental*, 1991. 17(30): 40–3.

20. H. J. Drew, et al. "Effect of Folate on Phenytoin Hyperplasia," *Journal of Clinical Periodontology*, 1987. 14: 350.

21. Sebastian G. Cianco, DDS, et al. Research presented to the International Association for Dental Research, 1994. Summarized in "Study Shows Mouthrinse Reduces Overgrowth of Gum Tissue," 1994. University of Buffalo: *http://www.buffalo.edu/scripts/newnews/studyshow8.html*.

22. Greg Krauss, MD, and Nathan Crone, MD. "Non-CNS Side Effects of Antiepileptic Drugs." *Neurology Treatment Updates*, 2000. Medscape, Inc.: *http://www.medscape.com/medscape/Neurology/TreatmentUpdate/2000/tu02/public/toc-tu02.html*.

Chapter 7, *Healthcare and Insurance*

1. Consumers for Quality Care, "HMO Arbitration Abuse Report." May 11, 2000: *http://www.consumerwatchdog.org/healthcare*.

Index

benzodiazepine tranquilizers, 146–147
See also specific names of medications
bibliographies, 231–235, 241, 244–245
biofeedback, 171–172
biotin, 178
bipolar disorders, 51, 186–187
birth defects, 77–78
black cohosh (Cimifuga racemosa), 183
black currant (Ribes nigrum), 183
blood tests, 38–39, 157–160, 188
board certification, 25
books, lists of, 231–235, 241, 244–245
brain
    communication within, 5–6
    damage to, 3
    degenerative disease as causes of
        seizures, 44–45
    diagrams of, 11, 14
    imaging, 36–38
    infections as causes of seizures,
        45–46, 165–166
    neurotransmitters in, 5–6
    as part of central nervous system,
        9–13
    structure and organization of, 9–13
    tumors/injury as causes of seizures,
        43–44
brain scans, 36–38
    preparation for, 38
    process, 36–37
    types of, 37–38
        BEAM (Brain Electrical
            Monitoring) EEG, 35
        CT/CAT (computerized
            tomography/computerized
            axial tomography), 37
        MRI (magnetic resonance
            imaging), 37–38
        PET (positron emission
            tomography), 38
        SPECT (single photon emission
            tomography), 38
breast feeding, 78–79, 152
breathing exercises, 170–171

C

calcium, 178
calcium channel blockers, 126–127

Canada
    disability income/financial support,
        84, 215–217
    responses to discrimination, 71
    single-payer healthcare, 23
Canadian Human Rights Act/
        Commission, 71
car insurance, 224–226
carbamazepine (Tegretol), 142–143
careers. *See* employment
carnitine, 180, 191
casein-free diet, 192
causes of seizures
    aging, 44–45, 48–49
    brain infections, 45–46, 165–166
    brain tumors/brain injury, 43–44
    degenerative brain disease, 44–45
    drug/supplement side effects, 46
    environmental triggers, 170-172
    hypoglycemia, 45
    stroke, 44–45, 49
    substance abuse, 47–48
    vascular abnormalities, 48–49
cavernomas, 49
cavernous angiomas, 49
cavernous malformations, 49
CBC (complete blood cell) count,
    159–160
central auditory processing disorder
    (CAPD), 52
central nervous system, 9–13
Cerebyx, 131–132
chamomile (Anthemis nobilis), 183
children and teens
    benign rolandic epilepsy, 4
    birth defects, 77–78
    counseling for, 174
    emotional maturity, 166
    and essential fatty acids, 186–187,
        189
    explaining seizures of, 119
    giving medication to, 150–152
    health insurance for, 23
    information needed by schools,
        67–68
    ongoing evaluation of, 166
    partial seizure disorders in, 4
    psychologists who work with, 28
    puberty, 166

children and teens (*continued*)
    respite care for, 119
    schools and Americans with
        Disabilities Act, 69
    sibling issues, 245
    social activities, 119–120
    sports, 120–121
    Temporary Assistance for Needy
        Families (TANF),
        213–214
    transition planning, 72
    transition to school after
        hospitalization, 110–111
    using steroids to treat, 147–149
    See also growing up with partial
        seizure disorders
Chinese medicine, 185
chiropractic adjustments, 171
chlordiazepoxide (Librium), 147
choline, 180
choosing specialists, 24–29
chromium picolinate, 179
clinical trials, 129, 224
clobazam (Frisium), 146
clonazepam (Klonopin), 137
clorazepate dipotassium (Tranxene), 147
combination educational settings, 107
comorbid conditions, 49
compassionate use laws, 129
complementary interventions/
        treatments. *See* non-
        medication measures
complex partial seizures, 3
compounding pharmacies, 150
controlling seizures. *See* stopping/
        shortening seizures
conversion disorder, 41
Convulex, 133–134
convulsions, 4
corticosteroids, 47, 54, 147–149
    See also hormones and hormonal
        disorders
counseling, 29, 173–175
CT/CAT (computerized tomography/
        computerized axial
        tomography) scan, 37

D

damiana (Turnera aphrodisiaca), 183
definitions of terms, 252–259
Delta-Cortef, 148
Deltasone, 148
denials of health insurance coverage/
        care. *See* health insurance
dental care, 192–193
Depakene, 132
Depakote, Depakote Sprinkles, 133–134
depression, 59–60
depth EEG, 35–36
developmental delays, 85–87
developmental disorders, 52
diabetes, 52–53
diagnosis
    difficulties with, 17–19
    by elimination (differential), 42–43
    general practitioner as team
        member, 26, 29
    of non-epileptic seizures, 41–42
    prognosis, 61
    recognizing partial seizures, 1-2
    report of, 60–61
    specialists needed for, 19–23
    team approach to, 26–29
    tests, 29–40
    waiting for, 60
    See also mimics of partial seizure
        disorders; specialists;
        tests, diagnostic
diagnostic classrooms, 103
Diamox, 134
diary of seizures, 20, 118, 247–248
Diazemuls, 147
diazepam (Valium), 147
diet and nutrition
    casein-free diet, 192
    effects on seizures, 189–190
    gluten-free diet, 192
    ketogenic diet, 124, 190–191, 241
    See also essential fatty acids;
        nutritional supplements;
        vitamins
differential diagnosis, 42–43
Dilantin, 134–135
discontinuing medication, 156–157

herbal remedies (*continued*)
    side effects of, 182–184
    specific
        black cohosh (Cimifuga
            racemosa), 183
        black currant (Ribes nigrum),
            183
        chamomile (Anthemis nobilis),
            183
        damiana (Turnera
            aphrodisiaca), 183
        gingko biloba, 183
        gotu kola (Centella asiatica,
            Hydrototyl asiatica), 183
        grapeseed oil, 183
        hops (Humulus lupulus), 183
        kava-kava (Piper
            methysticum), 183
        licorice (Glycyrrhiza glabra,
            Liquiritia officianalis), 184
        mistletoe (Viscum album), 184
        passion flower (Passiflora
            incarnata), 184
        Pycogenol, 183
        sarsaparilla (Hemidesmus
            indicus), 184
        skullcap (Scutellaria
            lateriflora), 184
        St. John's wort (Hypericum
            perforatum), 184
        valerian (Valeriana officinalis),
            184
HMOs. *See* health insurance
holistic approach to epilepsy
    as complementary intervention,
        168–169
    discussing with primary care
        doctor, 170
    and mainstream medicine, 167
    meaning of, 168
    specially trained providers, 167
homebound instruction, 105–106
homeschooling, 106
hops (Humulus lupulus), 183
hormones and hormonal disorders, 5–6,
    53–54
    See also steroids

hospital-based education, 105
hypoglycemia, 45

I

ictal, 9
IDEA (Individuals with Disabilities
    Education Act), 88–92
illegal drug use, 47–48, 152, 190
immune system research, 165–166
income support, 83–84
indirect financial help, 214–215
individual payment arrangements, 221
Individualized Education Plans (IEPs)
    accommodations, 94–97
    goals and objectives, 97–99
    meetings, 94
    overview of process, 92–93
    responses to refusal of schools to
        comply, 111–115
    signing/agreeing to, 99–100
    teens and self-advocacy, 93–94
Individualized Family Service Plan, 86
Individuals with Disabilities Education
    Act (IDEA), 88–92
infants. *See* children and teens
inositol, 180–181
insurance. *See* health insurance; auto
    insurance
inter-ictal, 9
intermittent explosive disorder (IED), 54
internet discussion groups, 24, 82–83
intracarotid sodium amobarbital (Wada)
    test, 39
Ireland, Republic of, benefits in,
    218–219

J

jobs. *See* employment
joint compression, 171
journal of seizures, 20, 118, 247–248

K

kava-kava (Piper methysticum), 183
Keppra, 136–137

ketogenic diet, 124, 167, 190–191, 241
kindling, 6–8, 187
Klonopin, 137

L

Lamictal, 138
lamotrigine (Lamictal), 138
laws and legal rights, 68–76
    504 plans, 69–70, 88–90
    Americans with Disabilities Act
        (ADA), 68–71
    Canadian Human Rights Act/
        Commission, 71
    compassionate use laws, 129
    driver's license guidelines, 80
    Equal Employment Opportunity
        Commission (US), 70
    Family and Medical Leave Act, 76
    Individuals with Disabilities
        Education Act (IDEA),
        88–92
    Rehabilitation Act of 1973 (US),
        70–71
    responses to discrimination
        in Canada, 71
        in the European Community,
        71
        in the United States, 71
    Social Security Disability Income
        (SSDI), 83–84
    Social Security Income (SSI), 83–84
    See also financial assistance; health
        insurance; schools and
        special education
lecithin, 181
leisure activities, 81
levetiracetam (Keppra), 136–137
Librium, 147
licorice (Glycyrrhiza glabra, Liquiritia
        officianalis), 184
life insurance, 224–226
lifestyle changes. See non-medication
        measures
limbic rage, 54
liver function/enzyme tests, 158–159

living with partial seizure disorders,
        62–84
    dealing with stigma, 63–65
    driving, 79–81
    employment, 72–76
    epilepsy awareness campaign, 64
    finding and building support,
        81–83
    income support, 81–83
    laws and legal rights, 68–76
    leisure activities, 81
    pregnancy, 76–79, 152
    responses to discrimination, 71–72
    seizures in public, 66–68
lorazepam (Ativan), 146
lumbar puncture, 39

M

managed care. See health insurance
manganese, 179
massage, 171
Matras, John
    "Trouble Afoot," 81
McLean hospital study, 186–187
medic alert bracelets and cards, 16, 68
medical insurance. See health insurance
medical interventions, 122–166
    anti-epilepsy drugs (AEDs),
        127–145
    benzodiazepine tranquilizers,
        146–147
    blood tests, 157–160
    drug level tests, 159–160
    electrocardiogram (EKG), 160
    finding a doctor, 125–126
    medications, generally
        discontinuing, 156–157
        drug interactions, 154–155
        eliminating/reducing costs of,
        222–224
        notes about, 149–152
        possible need for trying
            several, 4
        prescriptions, notes about, 154
        questions for doctor, 153

NeuroCybernetic Prosthesis, 160–162
neurologists, 4, 24
    See also specialists
neurology of seizures, 9–15
Neurontin, 138–139
neurotransmitters, 5–6
new and experimental treatments,
        165–166
New Zealand
    disability benefits, 84, 220–221
    health insurance, 220–221
    schools and special education,
        117–118
Nitrazadon, 139–140
nitrazepam (Nitrazadon), 139–140
non-epileptic seizures/pseudoseizures,
        41–42
non-medication measures, 124,
        167–195
    avoiding/managing environmental
        triggers, 170–172
    counseling, 29, 173–175
    dental care, 192–193
    diet and nutrition, 189–192
    essential fatty acids, 185–189
    hair and skin care, 193–194
    herbal remedies, 182–185
    holistic approach, 168–170
    minerals, 178–179
    need for care in using, 195
    not cures for epilepsy, 195
    nutritional supplements, 152,
        179–182
    positive mental attitude, 195
    stopping/shortening seizures, 173
    stress reduction, 170–172
    vitamins, 46, 175–178
notes, 249–251
nutrition. *See* diet and nutrition;
        essential fatty acids;
        nutritional supplements;
        vitamins
nutritional supplements, 152, 179–182
    carnitine, 180, 191
    choline, 180
    as foods, not drugs, 179
    GABA (gamma-aminobutyric acid),
        126–127, 180

inositol, 180–181
lecithin, 181
melatonin, 181
phenylalanine, 182
SAMe (s-adenosyl-methionine), 182
taurine, 181
tyrosine, 181
    See also essential fatty acids;
        vitamins
NutriVene-D, 189

O

occipital lobe, 12
Omega-3/Omega-6 fatty acids, 185
online discussion groups, 24, 82–83
Orasone, 148
Oriental medicine, 185
oxcarbazepine (Trileptal), 144

P

parietal lobe, 11–12, 12
partial seizure disorders, introduction to
    auras, 7–8, 51, 54–56
    brain damage as result of, 3
    causes, 2
    in children, 4
    control/prevention of, 4, 123–124
    defined, 1–2
    hormones and hormonal cycles,
        5–6, 53–54
    kindling, 6–8
    medical management of, 4
    neurology of, 9–15
    phases of seizures, 9
    physical and emotional effects of, 3
    recognizing, 1–2
    seizure focus, 2
    seizure threshold, 3
    terms, synonyms, and alternative
        names, 252–259
    types of partial seizures, 3–4
    what to do during seizures, 15–16
    in women, 5
passion flower (Passiflora incarnata),
        184
Peganone, 140

peri-ictal, 9
peripheral nervous system, 13–15
personality disorders, 56–58
    identified in/absent from DSM-IV, 56–58
    list/characteristics of, 57
    two ways of looking at, 56
PET (positron emission tomography) scan, 38
petit mal seizures, 4–5
pharmaceuticals. *See* medications
phases of seizures, 9
phenobarbital, 140–141
phenylalanine, 182
phenytoin (Dilantin), 134–135
physical effects of seizures, 3
physicians. *See* doctors; specialists
post-ictal, 9
prayer, 170
pre-ictal, 9
prednisolone (Prelone, Delta-Cortef), 148
prednisone (Deltasone, Orasone, Sterapred), 148
pregnancy
    birth defects, 77–78
    breast feeding, 78–79, 152
    minimizing AEDs during, 78
    seizures during, 76–79
    side effects of medications during, 152
Prelone, 148
prescriptions. *See* medications
primodone (Mysoline, Apo-Primidone, Myidone, Sertan), 148–149
private-pay arrangements, 221
private schools, 107
prodromal, 9
prognosis, 61
prolactin test, 39
pseudoseizures/non-epileptic seizures, 41–42
psychiatrists and psychologists, 26–29
psychological tests, 40
psychomotor seizures, 3
public, seizures in, 66–68
Pycogenol, 183

R

rages, 54
recognizing partial seizures, 1–2
referrals to/consultations with specialists, 19–25
Rehabilitation Act of 1973 (US), 70–71
releases of medical records, 20
repetitive Transcranial Magnetic Stimulation (rTMS), 165
Republic of Ireland, benefits in, 218
residential schools, 104
resources, 227–246
respite care, 119
Rimaprim, 147
Rivotril, 137

S

Sabril, 141–142
SAMe (s-adenosyl-methionine), 182
sarsaparilla (Hemidesmus indicus), 184
scalp EEG, 32
schizoaffective disorder, 58
schizophrenia, 58–59
schools and special education
    504 plans, 88–90
    alternative schools, 102–103
    in Australia, 117
    in Canada, 115–116
    combination settings, 107
    diagnostic classrooms, 103
    education mandated by law, 88
    finding out about, 87
    homebound instruction, 105–106
    homeschooling, 106
    hospital-based education, 105
    Individualized Education Plans (IEPs), 92–100
    Individuals with Disabilities Education Act (IDEA), 88–92
    informing schools of diagnosis, 87
    medications at, 109–110
    monitoring progress in, 108–109
    in New Zealand, 117–118
    placement decisions and options, 100, 107
    private schools, 107

steroids, 47, 54, 147–149
    See also hormones and hormonal
        disorders
stigma of partial seizure disorders,
    63–65, 65
    damage to self-esteem/
        embarrassment, 65
    discrimination, 64–65
    misunderstandings/attitudes toward
        epilepsy, 63–64
    need for self-advocacy, 65
Stoll, Andrew
    McLean hospital study, 186–187
stopping/shortening seizures
    with aromatherapy, 173
    with exercise, 173
    with food, 173
    role of diet in, 189–192
    with touch, 173
    See also stress reduction techniques
stress reduction techniques, 170–172
    acupuncture/acupressure, 172
    allergy reduction, 172
    breathing exercises, 170–171
    chiropractic adjustments, 171
    EEG biofeedback
        (neurobiofeedback),
        171–172
    joint compression, 171
    maintaining sleep schedules, 172
    massage, 171
    meditation, 170
    prayer, 170
stroke, 44–45, 49
subdural grid EEG, 36
substance abuse, 47–48, 152, 190
support
    finding and building, 81–83
    groups, list of, 227–230
surgery, 49, 162–164
syncope, 59

T

taking charge of treatment plan,
    124–125
TANF (Temporary Assistance for Needy
    Families), 213–214
taurine, 181

teens. *See* children and teens
Tegretol, 142–143
temporal lobe, 12
temporal lobe seizures/epilepsy, 3–5
Temporary Assistance for Needy
    Families (TANF),
    213–214
Tensium, 147
tests, diagnostic, 29–40
    blood, 38–39
    brain scans, 36–38
        preparation for, 38
        process, 36–37
        types of, 37–38
    electroencephalographs (EEGs), 17,
        31–36
        preparation for, 31–32
        process, 32
        reading results of, 32–33
        types of, 33–36
    at first meeting with neurologist,
        30–31
    genetic testing, 39–40, 233–234
    intracarotid sodium amobarbital
        (Wada), 39
    prolactin, 39
    psychological, 40
    spinal tap (lumbar puncture), 39
    See also diagnosis
therapy, 29, 173–175
tiagabine hydrochloride (Gabitril), 136
tobacco use, 152
tonic-clonic seizures, 4
Topamax, 143–144
topiramate (Topamax), 143–144
touch, preventing seizures with, 173
tranquilizers, 146–147
    See also specific names of medications
transportation services, 80, 239–240
Tranxene, 147
treatment goals
    making clear to doctors, 125–126
    seizure prevention, 123–124
treatment plan, 124–125
treatment teams, 26–29
TRICARE, 211
Trileptal, 144
Tropium, 147
"Trouble Afoot" (Matras), 81

About the Author

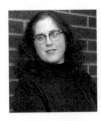

Mitzi Waltz is a journalist, a health researcher, and the parent of two children with special needs. She has authored four other books in O'Reilly's Patient-Centered Guides series, including *Pervasive Developmental Disorders: Finding a Diagnosis and Getting Help* and *Bipolar Disorders: A Guide to Helping Children and Adolescents*. Waltz is also an advocate for children with neurological and psychiatric disorders, and she is a PhD candidate at the University of Sunderland in England.

Colophon

Patient-Centered Guides are about the experience of illness. They contain personal stories as well as a combination of practical and medical information. The faces on the covers of our Guides reflect the human side of the information we offer.

The cover of *Partial Seizure Disorders: Help for Patients and Families* was designed by Terri Driscoll using Adobe Photoshop 5.5 and QuarkXPress 4.1 with Onyx BT and Berkeley fonts from Bitstream. The cover design is based on a series design by Edie Freedman. The cover photo is from Artville Stockimages and is used by permission.

The interior layout for the book was designed by Melanie Wang, based on a series design by Edie Freedman and Alicia Cech. The interior fonts are Berkeley and Franklin Gothic. Anne-Marie Vaduva prepared the text using FrameMaker 5.5.6. Illustrations were created by Robert Romano using Adobe Photoshop 5.5 and Macromedia Free-Hand 8.0

Catherine Morris was the production editor and copyeditor for *Partial Seizure Disorders: Help for Patients and Families*. Leanne Soylemez proofread the text, and Jeff Holcomb, Linley Dolby, and Claire Cloutier provided quality control. Kate Wilkinson wrote the index. Interior composition was done by Molly Shangraw and Catherine Morris.